AF107116

Copyright © 2024 by Sophia M. Johnson (Author)
All rights reserved. This book or any portion thereof may not be reproduced or used in any manner whatsoever without the express written permission of the publisher except for the use of brief quotations in a book review.
This book is copyright protected. This is only for personal use. You cannot amend, distributor, sell, use, quote or paraphrase any part or the content within this book without the consent of the author.
Please note the information contained within this document is for educational and entertainment purposes only. Every attempt has been made to provide accurate, up to date and reliable complete information. No warranties of any kind are expressed or implied. Readers acknowledge that the author is not engaging in the rendering of legal, financial, medical or professional advice. The content of this book has been derived from various sources. Please consult a licensed professional before attempting any techniques outlined in this book.
By reading this document, the readers agree that under no circumstances are the author responsible for any losses, direct or indirect, which are incurred as a result of the use of information contained within this document, including but not limited to errors, omissions or inaccuracies.

Thank you very much for reading this book.

Title: Clearing the Air: PM2.5, Health, and the Fight Against Pollution

Subtitle: A Deep Dive into the Impact of Air Pollution on Human Well-being and Global Efforts to Breathe Easy

Author: Sophia M. Johnson

Table of Contents

Introduction

Overview of PM2.5

In the invisible tapestry of our atmosphere, there exists a microscopic threat that has woven itself into the very air we breathe – PM2.5. Particulate Matter 2.5, abbreviated as PM2.5, represents particles with a diameter of 2.5 micrometers or smaller, invisible to the naked eye but wielding a profound impact on our health and environment. To embark on our journey through the pages of this book, it is crucial to gain a comprehensive understanding of this seemingly innocuous yet insidious pollutant.

PM2.5 particles originate from a myriad of sources, both natural and anthropogenic. Natural sources include wildfires, dust storms, and volcanic activities, releasing fine particles into the air. However, it is the human-driven activities that have significantly amplified the levels of PM2.5 globally. Combustion of fossil fuels, industrial processes, vehicular emissions, and agricultural practices all contribute to the release of these tiny particles into the atmosphere, creating a complex web of pollution that spans continents.

These particles, measuring a fraction of the width of a human hair, are adept at infiltrating the deepest recesses of our respiratory system. Unlike larger particles that get trapped in the nose or throat, PM2.5 can penetrate the lungs and even enter the bloodstream, posing serious health risks. The World Health Organization (WHO) identifies PM2.5 as a major environmental risk factor for a range of diseases, including respiratory and cardiovascular ailments. The implications of prolonged exposure to elevated PM2.5 levels are staggering, affecting not only the immediate well-being of individuals but also contributing to long-term health issues.

Understanding PM2.5 requires delving into the realms of atmospheric science and air quality monitoring. Advanced instruments and monitoring networks have been established worldwide to measure and analyze PM2.5 concentrations in real-time. These measurements provide a critical understanding of the spatial and temporal variations in PM2.5 levels, helping researchers and policymakers devise strategies to mitigate its impact.

As we progress through this exploration, it becomes evident that PM2.5 is not confined by borders. It transcends geographical boundaries, affecting urban and rural areas alike. The ubiquity of this pollutant underscores the urgent need for a collective and global response. Nations, communities, and individuals must unite in their efforts to address the pervasive issue of PM2.5 pollution.

In this book, we will unravel the multifaceted dimensions of PM2.5, examining its historical roots, global impact, repercussions on health, environmental consequences, and the concerted efforts being made to combat its proliferation. The journey begins with this comprehensive overview, a foundation upon which we will build our understanding of PM2.5 and its far-reaching implications. As we turn the pages, we will venture deeper into the intricate tapestry of air pollution, health, and the collective pursuit of cleaner, healthier air for all.

Importance of Addressing PM2.5 Pollution

The importance of addressing PM2.5 pollution extends far beyond the realm of environmental science; it penetrates the very fabric of human health, societal well-being, and the sustainable future of our planet. As we embark on this journey of exploration, it becomes imperative to unravel why PM2.5 has emerged as a critical focal point for researchers, policymakers, and concerned citizens alike.

At the heart of the matter lies the undeniable impact of PM2.5 on human health. These fine particles, minuscule in size but mighty in consequence, are capable of infiltrating the deepest recesses of the respiratory system. The human body, equipped to defend against larger particles, struggles to ward off the intrusion of PM2.5. Once inhaled, these particles can penetrate the lungs, enter the bloodstream, and wreak havoc on the cardiovascular system. The World Health Organization (WHO) identifies PM2.5 exposure as a leading cause of respiratory and cardiovascular diseases, contributing to millions of premature deaths globally.

The respiratory effects of PM2.5 are particularly alarming. Individuals exposed to elevated levels of PM2.5 may experience aggravated asthma, chronic bronchitis, and other respiratory ailments. Prolonged exposure can lead to reduced lung function, increased respiratory infections, and the development of more severe conditions such as lung cancer. The toll on cardiovascular health is equally concerning, with PM2.5 linked to an increased risk of heart attacks, strokes, and other cardiovascular diseases.

Moreover, the impact of PM2.5 pollution is not limited to individual health. It reverberates through communities, affecting vulnerable populations disproportionately. Children, the elderly, and individuals with pre-existing health conditions are more susceptible to the adverse effects of PM2.5, exacerbating existing health disparities. In this context, addressing PM2.5 pollution becomes a matter of environmental justice, with the burden of exposure falling disproportionately on marginalized communities.

Beyond health, PM2.5 pollution poses a substantial economic burden. The healthcare costs associated with treating illnesses caused or exacerbated by PM2.5 represent a significant drain on national economies. Lost productivity due to illness, medical expenses, and the societal costs of premature mortality all underscore the financial implications of neglecting the issue of PM2.5 pollution.

As we recognize the interconnectedness of human health and the environment, the importance of addressing PM2.5 pollution becomes paramount in the context of climate change. PM2.5 is not only a health hazard but also a potent climate-forcing agent. These particles can absorb and scatter sunlight, influencing local and regional climate patterns. The complex interplay between PM2.5 and climate change underscores the urgency of adopting strategies that not only improve air quality but also contribute to broader environmental sustainability goals.

On a global scale, PM2.5 pollution transcends borders. It is a shared challenge that necessitates international cooperation and coordinated efforts. The interconnected nature of our atmosphere means that the actions of one region can impact the air quality of another. As nations grapple with the consequences of a changing climate, addressing PM2.5 pollution emerges as a common ground for collaboration.

This brings us to the heart of our exploration – the importance of addressing PM2.5 pollution as a collective responsibility. The consequences of inaction are stark, with escalating health crises, economic burdens, and environmental degradation looming on the horizon. Recognizing the urgency, governments, organizations, and individuals around the world are increasingly turning their attention to comprehensive strategies aimed at reducing PM2.5 levels and safeguarding the well-being of current and future generations.

In the chapters that follow, we will delve deeper into the historical roots, global impact, health implications, environmental consequences, and the multifaceted efforts to combat PM2.5 pollution. The importance of addressing this pervasive challenge will resonate through every page, urging us to confront the complexities of air pollution and champion the cause of cleaner, healthier air for all.

Purpose: Unveiling the Layers of PM2.5

In the intricate tapestry of environmental challenges, this book emerges as a guide through the invisible but pervasive realm of PM2.5 pollution. As we navigate the chapters ahead, it is essential to illuminate the purpose and scope that drive our exploration, providing readers with a roadmap for the journey that lies ahead.

At the core of this endeavor is the purpose to demystify PM2.5, to peel back the layers of this microscopic antagonist and lay bare its intricacies. PM2.5, often relegated to the periphery of public awareness, demands our attention. This book aims to elevate PM2.5 from the shadows of obscurity, placing it under the spotlight for a comprehensive examination.

Our purpose extends beyond mere documentation; it is a call to action. By unraveling the complexities of PM2.5 pollution, we aspire to ignite a collective consciousness, fostering a shared responsibility for air quality. In doing so, we empower individuals, communities, and policymakers with the knowledge needed to confront this silent threat head-on.

Moreover, the purpose of this book is rooted in advocacy for change. We strive to be a catalyst for transformative action, urging stakeholders at every level to prioritize policies and practices that mitigate PM2.5 pollution. The urgency of this advocacy is underscored by the escalating health crises, environmental degradation, and the interconnected challenges of a changing climate.

Scope: Navigating the Dimensions of PM2.5

The scope of this book is expansive, mirroring the vast reach of PM2.5 pollution across geographical, ecological, and societal dimensions. We embark on a journey that spans the historical roots, global impact, health implications, environmental consequences, policy landscapes, technological innovations, public awareness efforts, and the future outlook of PM2.5 pollution.

Each chapter serves as a portal into a different facet of the PM2.5 narrative, allowing readers to delve into the historical evolution of awareness, witness the global consequences of this pollution, understand the intricacies of its impact on human health, explore the environmental repercussions, and grasp the nuanced interplay of policies and technological solutions.

The scope extends beyond the scientific to encompass the human element — the stories of communities affected, the advocacy efforts that shape policies, and the everyday choices that contribute to the broader narrative of air quality. By navigating this comprehensive scope, we aim to provide readers with a holistic understanding of PM2.5, recognizing that solutions must be as diverse and interconnected as the challenges themselves.

Moreover, the scope extends into the future, exploring emerging trends, challenges, and opportunities on the horizon. As we peer into the future chapters, we confront questions about the sustainability of our actions and the resilience of our ecosystems. The scope, therefore, is not merely retrospective but prospective, encouraging readers to contemplate the role they play in shaping a future where the air we breathe is cleaner and healthier.

In essence, the purpose and scope of this book converge on a singular objective — to illuminate the multifaceted dimensions of PM2.5 pollution and inspire informed, concerted efforts to address this global challenge. As we journey through the subsequent chapters, let us embark with a shared sense of purpose and an understanding of the expansive scope that lies before us.

Chapter 1: Historical Context

Early Awareness of Air Pollution

The awareness of air pollution, though now a prominent topic in environmental discourse, has its roots deeply embedded in the annals of history. Long before the advent of sophisticated monitoring systems and the recognition of specific pollutants like PM2.5, societies grappled with the tangible impacts of air quality degradation.

The Ancient Conundrum: A Haze Over Civilization

As early as ancient civilizations, individuals observed and grappled with the visible signs of air pollution. The burning of wood and other fuels for warmth and cooking released smoke into the air, creating a haze that blanketed early settlements. While these societies lacked the scientific vocabulary to describe pollutants, the consequences were evident – respiratory discomfort, eye irritation, and the visible presence of soot in the air.

In ancient Rome, for instance, the burning of coal for heating and cooking contributed to air pollution. The philosopher Seneca, in the first century AD, wrote about the impact of burning coal on the health of city dwellers. The nascent awareness of the connection between burning fuels and compromised air quality marks an early chapter in the acknowledgment of air pollution's presence.

Industrial Revolution: A Turning Point in Perception

The advent of the Industrial Revolution in the 18th century brought about a profound shift in the scale and nature of air pollution. The widespread use of coal-powered machinery and the expansion of industrial activities led to unprecedented emissions of pollutants into the atmosphere. In rapidly industrializing cities, the consequences became starkly apparent – smog-filled skies, respiratory illnesses, and a visible layer of soot on buildings.

One of the earliest documented instances of industrial air pollution impacting public health occurred in London during the 1952 Great Smog. The combustion of coal during a period of cold weather led to the formation of a dense smog that lingered over the city for several days. This event, which resulted in thousands of deaths and a surge in respiratory illnesses, prompted a reevaluation of the relationship between industrial activities and public health.

Air Pollution in the Pre-modern World: A Global Perspective

It is crucial to recognize that early awareness of air pollution was not confined to Western civilizations. In pre-modern China, for example, the burning of coal for heating and cooking contributed to air pollution in urban areas. Ancient Chinese texts reference the impact of this pollution on air quality and human health, reflecting an awareness that dates back centuries.

Similarly, in ancient India, where various forms of combustion were integral to daily life, early texts contain references to the impact of smoke on air quality. The Vedas, ancient Indian scriptures, acknowledge the importance of maintaining environmental balance and air purity.

The Emergence of Legislation: A Response to Early Crises

As awareness of air pollution grew, so did the need for regulatory measures. The mid-20th century witnessed the implementation of some of the world's first air quality regulations in response to severe pollution events. The Donora Smog of 1948 in Pennsylvania, USA, and the aforementioned Great Smog of London in 1952 prompted governments to take action.

These early crises underscored the need for systematic efforts to monitor and control air pollution. Legislation such as the Clean Air Act in the United States and the Clean Air Act of 1956 in the United Kingdom marked pivotal moments in the global recognition of air quality as a public health and environmental concern. These legislative responses set the stage for ongoing efforts to address air pollution on a broader scale.

As we traverse the historical landscape of early awareness of air pollution, it becomes evident that the seeds of concern were sown in the midst of smog-filled skies and the tangible impacts on human health. The historical context lays the groundwork for understanding how societies grappled with the visible signs of pollution and began to formulate responses that would shape the trajectory of environmental stewardship.

Evolution of Air Quality Metrics

In the pursuit of understanding and addressing air pollution, the evolution of air quality metrics stands as a testament to humanity's growing awareness of the intricate composition of our atmosphere. From the sooty skies of the Industrial Revolution to the establishment of systematic measurement methods, this chapter explores the historical journey of quantifying air quality.

The Early Observations: A Glimpse into Visible Pollution

Before the formalization of air quality metrics, societies relied on visible cues to assess the state of the air they breathed. The dense smog that enveloped industrializing cities during the 19th and early 20th centuries was a tangible sign of pollution. However, these early observations lacked precision, relying on subjective assessments of visibility and the presence of pollutants like soot.

The Birth of Monitoring Networks: Early Attempts to Quantify Pollution

The mid-20th century witnessed a paradigm shift with the establishment of monitoring networks and the introduction of rudimentary air quality measurements. Basic instruments capable of detecting particulate matter, sulfur dioxide, and other pollutants began to populate urban centers. This marked the first step towards quantifying air pollution in a systematic manner.

The inception of monitoring networks was often prompted by severe pollution events that captured public attention. Cities like Los Angeles, notorious for its smog, pioneered the implementation of monitoring stations to track pollutants and understand their sources. As these networks expanded, so did the realization that a more nuanced understanding of air quality required a broader set of metrics.

From Visible to Invisible: The Advent of Particulate Matter Metrics

While early air quality monitoring focused on visible pollutants like soot and sulfur dioxide, the realization that not all harmful particles were visible to the naked eye prompted the development of more sophisticated metrics. Particulate matter, particularly PM10 (particles with a diameter of 10 micrometers or smaller), became a key metric as researchers sought to quantify the diverse range of particles suspended in the air.

As scientific understanding advanced, it became evident that even finer particles, specifically those with a diameter of 2.5 micrometers or smaller (PM2.5), posed significant health risks. The evolution of air quality metrics thus shifted towards the inclusion of finer particulate matter measurements, marking a pivotal moment in the quest for a comprehensive understanding of airborne pollutants.

The Birth of Air Quality Indices: Simplifying Complexity for Public Awareness

As air quality metrics grew more sophisticated, the challenge arose of translating complex data into understandable information for the general public. The development of Air Quality Indices (AQI) addressed this challenge by providing a simplified numerical scale to communicate the overall air quality to the public. The AQI considers multiple pollutants, including PM2.5, ozone, sulfur dioxide, nitrogen dioxide, and carbon monoxide, amalgamating them into a single, easily interpretable value.

The introduction of AQI not only facilitated public awareness but also became a crucial tool for policymakers in crafting targeted interventions. It allowed for the categorization of air quality into different levels, each associated with recommended actions to protect public health. This standardized approach enabled a more consistent evaluation of air quality on a national and international scale.

Globalization of Air Quality Metrics: Harmonizing Standards

As air pollution became recognized as a transboundary issue, the need for standardized metrics and monitoring approaches became apparent. International collaborations led to the establishment of common frameworks and standards for air quality measurement, ensuring consistency in reporting and facilitating global comparisons.

The World Health Organization (WHO), in collaboration with other international bodies, played a pivotal role in developing global guidelines for air quality. These guidelines not only set thresholds for pollutants but also underscored the importance of considering the cumulative impact of multiple pollutants on human health. The harmonization of air quality metrics became an essential step in addressing the interconnected challenges posed by air pollution.

Technological Advancements: Precision in Monitoring

Advancements in technology have revolutionized air quality monitoring, offering unprecedented precision and real-time data. Remote sensing, satellite technology, and sophisticated monitoring instruments provide a more comprehensive and dynamic understanding of air quality patterns. These technological leaps enable researchers to track pollutants at finer spatial scales, identify pollution hotspots, and assess the effectiveness of mitigation strategies with greater accuracy.

The evolution of air quality metrics reflects a profound journey from subjective observations of sooty skies to the sophisticated, data-driven approaches of the present day. As we navigate through the historical context, the progression from visible pollution to the quantifiable metrics of PM2.5 and AQI marks a crucial chapter in our collective efforts to comprehend, measure, and ultimately address the complexities of air pollution.

Emergence of PM2.5 as a Significant Indicator

In the annals of air quality history, a microscopic protagonist emerged from the haze to claim its place as a significant indicator — PM2.5. This chapter delves into the historical journey that elevated PM2.5 from an obscure particle to a critical metric in understanding and addressing air pollution.

The Invisible Culprit: Unmasking Fine Particulate Matter

As early air quality monitoring networks took root in the mid-20th century, the focus primarily rested on visible pollutants such as soot and sulfur dioxide. However, the realization dawned that not all harmful particles were discernible to the naked eye. Enter PM2.5 — particulate matter with a diameter of 2.5 micrometers or smaller.

PM2.5 represented a new frontier in air quality assessment. Unlike larger particles that could be trapped by the body's natural defenses, PM2.5 had the ability to penetrate deep into the respiratory system. This unique characteristic, combined with its ubiquity in various pollution sources, hinted at a more insidious threat to human health than previously acknowledged.

Early Research: Tracing the Health Impacts of PM2.5

Scientific inquiry into the health impacts of PM2.5 began to gain traction in the latter half of the 20th century. Early studies, though limited in scope, hinted at a correlation between elevated levels of fine particulate matter and adverse health effects. The ability of PM2.5 to reach the lower respiratory tract and even enter the bloodstream raised concerns among researchers and health professionals.

The landmark Harvard Six Cities Study, conducted in the 1990s, provided crucial insights into the long-term health effects of PM2.5 exposure. The study, which spanned multiple U.S. cities, demonstrated a clear association between elevated levels of fine particulate matter and increased mortality rates, particularly from cardiovascular and respiratory diseases. These findings served as a catalyst for recognizing PM2.5 as a significant indicator of health risks.

Regulatory Response: Integrating PM2.5 into Air Quality Standards

The growing body of evidence on the health impacts of PM2.5 spurred regulatory bodies to revisit and refine air quality standards. The United States Environmental Protection Agency (EPA), for instance, incorporated PM2.5 into the National Ambient Air Quality Standards (NAAQS) in 1997. This marked a pivotal moment in recognizing the unique risks posed by fine particulate matter and the need for targeted regulations to curb its levels.

Internationally, the World Health Organization (WHO) followed suit, providing guidelines for PM2.5 concentrations and emphasizing the importance of limiting exposure to protect public health. The inclusion of PM2.5 as a specific indicator in air quality standards represented a paradigm shift, acknowledging the distinct threat posed by these fine particles.

Technological Advancements: Precision in PM2.5 Monitoring

The integration of PM2.5 into air quality standards paralleled advancements in monitoring technology. Traditional monitoring methods, which primarily focused on larger particles, needed augmentation to capture the finer nuances of PM2.5 pollution. High-precision instruments capable of detecting and quantifying PM2.5 levels with accuracy became essential tools in the fight against this invisible adversary.

Satellite technology and remote sensing further enhanced our ability to monitor PM2.5 on a global scale. These technological advancements not only improved the accuracy of measurements but also provided a more comprehensive understanding of the spatial and temporal patterns of PM2.5 pollution. This newfound precision was crucial for devising targeted strategies to mitigate the impact of fine particulate matter on air quality.

Public Awareness: From Obscurity to Prominence

As PM2.5 took its place as a significant indicator of air quality, efforts were made to raise public awareness about this invisible threat. Public health campaigns, environmental organizations, and educational initiatives sought to communicate the risks associated with PM2.5 exposure. The integration of PM2.5 data into Air Quality Indices (AQI), accessible to the general public, further facilitated understanding and underscored the importance of monitoring and addressing fine particulate matter.

Global Recognition: PM2.5 as a Cross-Border Concern

The international community began to recognize PM2.5 not merely as a local or national issue but as a global concern.

The interconnected nature of air masses meant that elevated PM2.5 levels in one region could impact air quality in distant locations. Collaborative efforts to address cross-border air pollution required a common understanding of the significance of PM2.5 as a shared metric.

International organizations, including the United Nations and regional environmental bodies, emphasized the need for harmonized approaches to PM2.5 monitoring and regulation. Global initiatives aimed at reducing fine particulate matter emissions gained momentum, reflecting a collective acknowledgment of the importance of PM2.5 as a transboundary pollutant.

Challenges and Ongoing Research: Unraveling the Complexities

Despite the strides made in understanding and addressing PM2.5, challenges persist. Ongoing research endeavors seek to unravel the complexities of fine particulate matter, exploring the sources, transformation processes, and regional variations in PM2.5 composition. The dynamic nature of PM2.5 pollution necessitates continual advancements in monitoring technology and a nuanced understanding of the factors influencing its distribution and impact.

As we reflect on the historical emergence of PM2.5 as a significant indicator, it becomes evident that this journey is not confined to the past. The ongoing evolution of research, regulations, and technological capabilities highlights the enduring importance of PM2.5 in the broader context of air quality management. PM2.5, once an invisible threat lurking in the haze, now stands as a beacon guiding our collective efforts to breathe cleaner, healthier air.

Historical Incidents and Case Studies

In the historical narrative of air quality, specific incidents and case studies serve as poignant chapters, revealing the tangible and sometimes devastating impact of PM2.5 on human health, the environment, and communities. This section delves into these historical incidents, providing insights into the complexities and consequences of elevated PM2.5 levels.

The Great Smog of London (1952): A Lethal Blanket of Fog

One of the most notorious events in the history of air pollution, the Great Smog of London in 1952, stands as a stark reminder of the lethal consequences of elevated PM2.5 levels. A combination of cold weather, windless conditions, and widespread coal burning led to the formation of a thick smog that engulfed the city for several days.

What appeared as an ordinary fog harbored an invisible menace – elevated concentrations of pollutants, including PM2.5. The smog contributed to respiratory issues and other health problems, leading to an estimated 4,000 additional deaths. This tragic event became a catalyst for reevaluating air quality standards and spurred regulatory actions to address the impact of pollution on public health.

The Donora Smog (1948): An Early Warning

In 1948, the small town of Donora in Pennsylvania, USA, experienced a deadly smog event that foreshadowed the broader implications of air pollution. Industrial emissions, including particulate matter, became trapped in a temperature inversion, creating a stagnant layer of polluted air over the town. The result was a severe smog that persisted for several days.

The Donora Smog is associated with increased mortality and respiratory illnesses, highlighting the acute health effects of elevated PM2.5 levels. This incident, though localized, drew attention to the potential dangers of industrial pollution and contributed to the growing awareness of the need for regulatory measures to protect public health.

The Meuse Valley Fog (1930): Early Recognition of Health Impacts

The Meuse Valley fog event in 1930, in Belgium, is often considered one of the earliest instances where the health impacts of air pollution were recognized. A temperature inversion trapped industrial emissions, leading to a dense fog with elevated concentrations of pollutants, including sulfur dioxide and particulate matter.

This incident resulted in a significant number of deaths and hospital admissions due to respiratory and cardiovascular issues. The Meuse Valley fog underscored the correlation between air pollution and adverse health effects, contributing to a gradual shift in public perception and scientific understanding of the link between atmospheric conditions, pollution, and health.

Asian Brown Cloud: A Modern Regional Challenge

In more recent times, the Asian Brown Cloud has emerged as a prominent case study illustrating the regional and global implications of air pollution, including elevated levels of PM2.5. This large-scale atmospheric phenomenon, characterized by the presence of a widespread brownish haze, spans across parts of Asia and the Indian Ocean.

The Asian Brown Cloud is a complex interplay of natural and anthropogenic factors, with particulate matter, including PM2.5, playing a significant role. The cloud has been linked to adverse health effects, regional climate impacts, and the deposition of pollutants over distant areas. This case study highlights the interconnectedness of air quality issues on a continental scale.

Mexico City Air Quality Crisis: Urban Challenges

Mexico City has faced persistent air quality challenges, epitomized by recurring episodes of high PM2.5 levels. The combination of rapid urbanization, vehicular emissions, and geographical factors has contributed to elevated levels of fine particulate matter. The city's topography, surrounded by mountains, often traps pollutants, exacerbating air quality issues.

The Mexico City case study emphasizes the complexity of managing air quality in densely populated urban areas, where multiple pollution sources converge. Efforts to address the PM2.5 crisis in Mexico City involve a combination of regulatory measures, public awareness campaigns, and technological innovations aimed at mitigating the impact of air pollution on the city's residents.

Lessons from Historical Incidents: A Call to Action

These historical incidents and case studies underscore the urgency of addressing elevated PM2.5 levels. Beyond the statistics lie the stories of communities grappling with the immediate and long-term consequences of air pollution. These incidents have left an indelible mark on the trajectory of environmental policy, prompting regulatory actions, technological innovations, and a collective recognition of the need to protect air quality for current and future generations.

As we reflect on these historical chapters, they serve as a call to action. The lessons learned from events like the Great Smog of London, the Donora Smog, the Meuse Valley fog, the Asian Brown Cloud, and the Mexico City air quality crisis propel us towards a future where proactive measures, international cooperation, and technological advancements can mitigate the impact of PM2.5 and ensure a healthier, cleaner environment for all.

Chapter 2: Global Impact

PM2.5 as a Global Environmental Challenge

The pervasive presence of PM2.5 transcends geographical boundaries, making it a formidable global environmental challenge. This chapter explores the interconnected nature of PM2.5 pollution, delving into its transboundary impact, environmental consequences, and the shared responsibility of the international community in addressing this invisible menace.

The Atmospheric Wanderer: Understanding the Transboundary Movement of PM2.5

PM2.5, with its minuscule size and weight, possesses a unique ability to travel vast distances through the atmosphere. The atmospheric currents, prevailing winds, and weather patterns become conduits for the global dissemination of these fine particles. As a result, PM2.5 emitted in one region can influence air quality and environmental conditions in distant areas.

Studies utilizing satellite observations and atmospheric modeling have elucidated the transboundary movement of PM2.5. Emissions from industrial activities, wildfires, and anthropogenic sources can disperse particles across continents. This phenomenon underscores the need for a collaborative, international approach to address the complexities of PM2.5 pollution.

Global Hotspots: Identifying Regions of Elevated PM2.5 Levels

While PM2.5 can disperse widely, certain regions emerge as global hotspots, experiencing consistently elevated levels of fine particulate matter. These hotspots are often characterized by a combination of factors, including industrial emissions, urbanization, geographical features, and meteorological conditions that trap pollutants.

Parts of Asia, including India and China, are recognized as significant global hotspots for PM2.5 pollution. Rapid industrialization, dense urban populations, and agricultural activities contribute to elevated levels of fine particulate matter in the atmosphere. However, hotspots are not confined to specific continents; localized sources and regional factors can create pockets of heightened PM2.5 levels globally.

The Arctic Paradox: PM2.5 in Pristine Environments

Even remote, seemingly pristine environments, such as the Arctic, are not immune to the influence of PM2.5 pollution. The phenomenon known as the Arctic haze involves the transport of pollutants, including fine particulate matter, to the Arctic region from distant sources. This paradoxical contamination highlights the interconnectedness of the global atmosphere and the far-reaching impact of human activities on even the most remote ecosystems.

The presence of PM2.5 in the Arctic has implications for the delicate balance of Arctic ecosystems and wildlife. The deposition of pollutants in snow and ice can accelerate melting, affecting sea ice dynamics and contributing to broader climate change concerns. The Arctic serves as a poignant reminder that addressing PM2.5 pollution requires a holistic understanding of its global reach and diverse environmental consequences.

Health Impacts on a Global Scale: PM2.5 and Respiratory Diseases

The transboundary nature of PM2.5 extends beyond environmental consequences to impact global public health. Elevated levels of fine particulate matter have been linked to an increased prevalence of respiratory diseases on a global scale. The inhalation of PM2.5 particles, capable of penetrating deep into the respiratory system, poses health risks for individuals across continents.

Research indicates that exposure to elevated levels of PM2.5 is associated with a higher incidence of respiratory conditions, including asthma, chronic bronchitis, and lung cancer. Vulnerable populations, such as children, the elderly, and individuals with pre-existing health conditions, are particularly susceptible to the health impacts of PM2.5, emphasizing the need for a concerted international effort to mitigate the global burden of respiratory diseases.

Global Economic Costs: The Toll of PM2.5 on Productivity and Healthcare

The global impact of PM2.5 is not confined to environmental and health realms but extends to economic consequences. The healthcare costs associated with treating respiratory and cardiovascular diseases linked to PM2.5 exposure impose a substantial economic burden on nations around the world. Beyond healthcare expenditures, the productivity losses resulting from illness and premature mortality further underscore the economic toll of PM2.5 pollution.

A study by the World Bank estimated that the global economic costs of air pollution, including PM2.5, amount to trillions of dollars annually. These costs encompass medical expenses, reduced labor productivity, and the broader socio-economic ramifications of air pollution-related health crises. The recognition of the economic toll adds another layer of urgency to the need for coordinated global efforts to address PM2.5 pollution.

International Initiatives: Collaborative Strategies to Tackle PM2.5

Recognizing the global nature of PM2.5 pollution, international initiatives and collaborations have emerged to address this shared environmental challenge. Organizations such as the United Nations Environment Programme (UNEP), the World Health Organization (WHO), and regional bodies work towards establishing common frameworks, guidelines, and targets for addressing PM2.5 levels.

The Sustainable Development Goals (SDGs), particularly Goal 3 (Good Health and Well-being) and Goal 11 (Sustainable Cities and Communities), underscore the importance of tackling air pollution, including PM2.5, as a component of broader global development objectives. The Paris Agreement on climate change also acknowledges the interlinkages between air quality, climate, and health, emphasizing the need for comprehensive strategies to address PM2.5 pollution.

Technological Innovation: Global Solutions for Global Challenges

In the quest to tackle PM2.5 pollution on a global scale, technological innovation plays a pivotal role. Advancements in monitoring technology, satellite observations, and data-sharing platforms enable real-time tracking of PM2.5 levels worldwide. These tools facilitate the identification of hotspots, the assessment of regional trends, and the evaluation of the effectiveness of mitigation measures.

Technological innovation extends beyond monitoring to encompass cleaner technologies, emission control devices, and sustainable urban planning. Collaborative research and development initiatives foster the exchange of knowledge and best practices, allowing nations to leapfrog to cleaner, more sustainable solutions and reduce their reliance on PM2.5-emitting technologies.

The Urgency of Global Action: A Call for Collective Responsibility

As PM2.5 continues to impact air quality, environmental health, and communities worldwide, the urgency of global action becomes increasingly evident. The interconnectedness of the global atmosphere mandates a collective responsibility to address the transboundary impact of PM2.5 pollution. Nations must collaborate to share data, implement effective policies, and invest in sustainable practices that reduce PM2.5 emissions.

The global environmental challenge posed by PM2.5 demands a paradigm shift in how societies approach air quality management. From regional hotspots to the farthest reaches of the Arctic, the impact of PM2.5 on ecosystems, human health, and the economy requires holistic, cooperative solutions. In the chapters that follow, we will explore the nuanced strategies, success stories, and ongoing challenges in the global quest to mitigate the impact of PM2.5 pollution and secure a healthier future for our planet.

Regional Variances in PM2.5 Levels

As we explore the global impact of PM2.5 pollution, it becomes evident that the distribution of fine particulate matter is not uniform across the planet. Regional variances in PM2.5 levels paint a complex tapestry influenced by geographical, meteorological, and anthropogenic factors. This chapter delves into the intricacies of regional disparities, examining the hotspots, challenges, and unique dynamics that shape PM2.5 concentrations on a continental scale.

Asia: The Epicenter of PM2.5 Hotspots

The Asian continent emerges as a focal point for elevated PM2.5 levels, hosting some of the world's most notorious hotspots for fine particulate matter pollution. Rapid industrialization, urbanization, and a burgeoning population contribute to the concentration of PM2.5 in several Asian countries.

India: India, with its diverse landscapes and industrial hubs, experiences significant regional variances in PM2.5 levels. Urban centers like Delhi, Kolkata, and Mumbai often grapple with elevated concentrations attributed to vehicular emissions, industrial activities, and agricultural practices. The Indo-Gangetic Plain, surrounded by the Himalayas, frequently witnesses atmospheric conditions that trap pollutants, exacerbating PM2.5 levels.

China: China, another major contributor to global PM2.5 levels, faces substantial regional disparities. Industrialized regions such as the Pearl River Delta and the Yangtze River Delta exhibit higher concentrations due to industrial emissions, coal combustion, and urbanization. Geographic features, including mountain ranges, can influence the dispersion and accumulation of PM2.5, contributing to variability across different provinces.

Southeast Asia: Southeast Asian nations, including Indonesia, Malaysia, and Thailand, contend with PM2.5 challenges arising from agricultural activities, deforestation, and biomass burning. The annual haze episodes, often driven by the intentional burning of forests for agricultural purposes, elevate PM2.5 levels in the region, impacting air quality and posing health risks.

North America: Urban Centers and Industrial Regions

In North America, regional variances in PM2.5 levels are influenced by a combination of urbanization, industrial activities, and geographical features. While overall air quality has improved in recent decades due to regulatory measures, certain areas continue to face challenges.

United States: Urban centers and industrial regions in the United States, such as Los Angeles, the Midwest, and the Northeast, experience elevated PM2.5 levels. Traffic-related emissions, industrial processes, and seasonal factors contribute to regional disparities. The western part of the country, with its expansive deserts and less industrialized areas, generally exhibits lower PM2.5 concentrations.

Canada: Canada's regional disparities in PM2.5 levels are influenced by industrial activities, transportation, and natural sources. Urban centers like Toronto and Vancouver may face localized challenges, while remote areas benefit from lower population density and fewer anthropogenic emissions. The Arctic regions of Canada, despite their pristine environment, are not immune to the long-range transport of PM2.5.

Europe: Urbanization, Industrialization, and Transboundary Transport

Europe, with its diverse mix of urban and rural landscapes, grapples with regional variances in PM2.5 levels shaped by industrialization, urbanization, and the transport of pollutants across national borders.

Western Europe: Industrialized regions in Western Europe, including parts of the United Kingdom, Germany, and France, face challenges associated with PM2.5 emissions from industrial sources, transportation, and residential combustion. Urban centers with high population density, such as London and Paris, may experience elevated concentrations.

Eastern Europe: Eastern European nations, transitioning from centrally planned to market-oriented economies, encounter unique challenges in managing PM2.5 levels. Legacy issues, including outdated industrial infrastructure, contribute to regional disparities. The transboundary transport of pollutants further influences air quality in this region.

Latin America: Urbanization and Biomass Burning

Latin American countries contend with regional variations in PM2.5 levels influenced by urbanization, industrial activities, and the widespread practice of biomass burning.

Mexico: Mexico, characterized by rapid urbanization and industrialization, faces elevated PM2.5 levels in major urban centers like Mexico City and Monterrey. Vehicular emissions, industrial processes, and topographical features contribute to regional disparities.

Brazil: The vast Amazon rainforest in Brazil, while acting as a global lung, experiences seasonal challenges associated with biomass burning. The intentional clearing of land for agriculture contributes to elevated PM2.5 levels during certain periods, impacting air quality in both rural and urban areas.

Africa: Urbanization, Industrialization, and Natural Sources

Africa, with its diverse ecosystems and rapidly growing urban centers, grapples with regional disparities in PM2.5 levels influenced by urbanization, industrialization, and natural sources.

North Africa: Urban centers in North Africa, including Cairo and Casablanca, may experience elevated PM2.5 levels due to industrial emissions, traffic-related pollution, and geographical factors. Dust storms, prevalent in arid regions, contribute to particulate matter concentrations.

Sub-Saharan Africa: Rapid urbanization and industrialization in some sub-Saharan African countries lead to localized challenges in managing PM2.5 levels. Natural sources, such as dust storms and wildfires, also influence regional disparities in air quality.

Oceania: Urban Centers and Natural Influences

Oceania, encompassing Australia and the Pacific Islands, exhibits regional variances in PM2.5 levels influenced by urbanization, industrial activities, and natural sources.

Australia: Major urban centers in Australia, including Sydney and Melbourne, may face elevated PM2.5 levels due to urban and industrial emissions. The country also experiences episodes of bushfires, contributing to short-term increases in fine particulate matter.

Pacific Islands: Remote Pacific Islands generally have lower PM2.5 levels, benefiting from lower population density and limited industrialization. However, regional influences, such as biomass burning or transboundary transport, can contribute to localized challenges.

Antarctica: A Pristine Environment at Risk

Even the pristine continent of Antarctica is not immune to the global reach of PM2.5. Although sparsely populated, research stations and human activities contribute to localized challenges. Long-range transport of pollutants, including fine particulate matter, can impact the air quality in this remote region and pose risks to the delicate Antarctic ecosystem.

Factors Influencing Regional Variances

Several factors contribute to the regional disparities in PM2.5 levels observed across continents:

1. Anthropogenic Sources: The concentration of industrial activities, vehicular emissions, and energy production can significantly influence regional PM2.5 levels. Urbanization and population density also play a crucial role.

2. Natural Sources: Natural events such as dust storms, wildfires, and volcanic eruptions contribute to fluctuations in PM2.5 levels. Geographical features and climatic conditions influence the prevalence of these natural sources.

3. Meteorological Conditions: Atmospheric conditions, including temperature inversions and prevailing winds, can impact the dispersion and accumulation of PM2.5. Certain regions may experience stagnation of air masses, leading to elevated concentrations.

4. Regulatory Measures: The effectiveness of air quality regulations and enforcement varies globally, influencing the success of mitigation efforts. Regions with stringent regulatory frameworks may experience better air quality compared to areas with lax enforcement.

5. Socioeconomic Factors: The level of economic development, access to clean technologies, and socioeconomic disparities contribute to regional variations in PM2.5 levels. Developed regions may have resources to invest in cleaner technologies, while developing areas may face challenges in implementing mitigation measures.

Addressing Regional Disparities: A Call for Comprehensive Strategies

As we navigate the complex tapestry of regional variances in PM2.5 levels, it becomes clear that addressing this global environmental challenge requires comprehensive strategies tailored to the unique dynamics of each region. Collaborative efforts, international cooperation, and the sharing of best practices can facilitate the development and implementation of effective mitigation measures.

In the chapters that follow, we will delve into specific case studies, success stories, and ongoing challenges in diverse regions, aiming to unravel the intricacies of managing PM2.5 pollution on a continental scale. The journey towards cleaner air involves not only understanding the factors contributing to regional disparities but also fostering a collective commitment to safeguarding the global atmosphere for generations to come.

Impact on Urban and Rural Areas

As PM2.5 pollution pervades the global atmosphere, its impact unfolds in a nuanced dichotomy, affecting both urban and rural areas with distinct challenges and consequences. This chapter explores the intricate dynamics of how fine particulate matter shapes the air quality landscape in urban centers and rural landscapes, unraveling the dual face of PM2.5's influence on diverse communities.

Urban Areas: Breathing in the Shadows of Progress

Urbanization, marked by the rapid growth of cities and the concentration of population and industries, amplifies the challenges posed by PM2.5 pollution in urban areas.

Air Quality Hotspots: Urban centers worldwide grapple with elevated PM2.5 levels, often surpassing air quality standards. Traffic congestion, industrial emissions, and dense human activities contribute to localized hotspots where fine particulate matter concentrations soar. Cities like Beijing, New Delhi, and Cairo have become synonymous with the visible haze of PM2.5, casting shadows over the skylines.

Health Impacts in Urban Populations: The dense populations of urban areas expose a significant number of people to the health risks associated with PM2.5 exposure. Respiratory diseases, cardiovascular ailments, and increased mortality rates are prevalent health impacts. Vulnerable groups, including children and the elderly, face heightened susceptibility, leading to a public health crisis that demands urgent attention.

Economic Consequences: Urban economies bear the brunt of PM2.5 pollution through increased healthcare expenditures, productivity losses, and impacts on the overall quality of life. The economic toll extends to medical costs, absenteeism, and reduced labor productivity, affecting the prosperity of urban communities.

Social Inequities: Within urban settings, social inequities exacerbate the impact of PM2.5 pollution. Marginalized communities often reside in proximity to industrial zones and traffic corridors, experiencing disproportionately higher levels of exposure. This environmental injustice deepens existing social disparities, underscoring the need for inclusive policies that address the unequal burden of PM2.5 pollution.

Mitigation Challenges: The complex urban landscape poses challenges for mitigating PM2.5 pollution. Balancing the demand for economic growth with environmental sustainability is a delicate task. Implementing effective measures, such as transitioning to cleaner technologies, improving public transportation, and enhancing green spaces, requires collaborative efforts between government bodies, industries, and the urban populace.

Rural Areas: Echoes of Agriculture and Natural Sources

While urban areas grapple with the visible impact of industrialization, rural landscapes face their own set of challenges influenced by agricultural practices, biomass burning, and natural sources of PM2.5.

Agricultural Contributions: Rural regions are often characterized by extensive agricultural activities, including crop cultivation and livestock farming. Agricultural practices, such as the use of fertilizers and pesticides, contribute to the release of particulate matter into the air. Dust from tilled fields and unpaved roads further adds to the PM2.5 burden in rural areas.

Biomass Burning: Traditional cooking methods, reliance on solid fuels, and seasonal practices like crop residue burning contribute to elevated PM2.5 levels in rural areas. The combustion of biomass releases fine particulate matter, affecting both air quality and the health of communities reliant on these practices.

Indoor Air Quality: While urban areas often grapple with outdoor air pollution, rural communities face challenges related to indoor air quality. The use of traditional stoves and open fires for cooking and heating exposes inhabitants to high concentrations of PM2.5 within their homes. Indoor air pollution becomes a significant health concern, particularly for women and children who spend extended periods indoors.

Health Impacts in Rural Populations: The health consequences of PM2.5 exposure extend to rural populations, albeit with unique dimensions. Respiratory ailments, cardiovascular diseases, and adverse pregnancy outcomes are prevalent health concerns. Limited access to healthcare facilities in rural areas exacerbates the vulnerability of communities facing the dual burden of indoor and outdoor PM2.5 pollution.

Economic Dependence on Agriculture: Rural economies, often reliant on agriculture, face economic repercussions due to PM2.5 pollution. Crop yield reductions, livestock health issues, and the overall environmental degradation influence the livelihoods of rural communities. Sustainable agricultural practices and clean energy solutions become pivotal for mitigating the economic impact of PM2.5 pollution.

Community Resilience and Education: Building resilience in rural communities involves not only implementing clean energy solutions but also fostering awareness and education. Empowering communities to understand the sources and health impacts of PM2.5 pollution enables proactive measures. Community-led initiatives, sustainable farming practices, and the promotion of clean cooking technologies contribute to building resilience in the face of environmental challenges.

The Interconnected Reality: Urban-Rural Linkages

The impact of PM2.5 pollution blurs the boundaries between urban and rural areas, creating linkages that underscore the interconnected reality of air quality challenges.

Urban-Rural Migration: The migration of individuals from rural to urban areas, driven by economic opportunities, exacerbates the challenges associated with PM2.5 pollution. Urbanization intensifies as populations concentrate in cities, leading to increased demand for resources and energy, and subsequently, higher emissions of fine particulate matter.

Agricultural-Urban Nexus: The nexus between urban demand for agricultural products and rural farming practices creates a cycle of PM2.5 pollution. The use of fertilizers and pesticides in rural areas, driven by the demand for food in urban centers, contributes to outdoor air pollution. Similarly, the combustion of biomass for cooking in rural households is influenced by urban energy consumption patterns.

Climate Change Interactions: PM2.5 pollution interacts with broader environmental issues, including climate change. The influence of fine particulate matter on regional climates can affect both urban and rural areas. In turn, changing climatic conditions impact the dispersion and transport of PM2.5, creating a feedback loop that requires holistic strategies for mitigation and adaptation.

Mitigation Strategies: Tailoring Approaches to Diverse Landscapes

Addressing the dual impact of PM2.5 pollution in both urban and rural areas necessitates tailored mitigation strategies that account for the unique challenges and dynamics of each landscape.

Urban Solutions:

- Clean Transportation: Transitioning to electric vehicles, improving public transportation, and promoting sustainable urban planning contribute to reducing vehicular emissions in urban areas.

- Green Infrastructure: Increasing green spaces, implementing urban forestry initiatives, and creating parks help absorb pollutants and enhance air quality in cities.

- Industrial Upgrades: Encouraging industries to adopt cleaner technologies, implement emission controls, and adhere to stringent air quality standards is crucial for mitigating PM2.5 pollution in urban centers.

Rural Solutions:

- Clean Cooking Technologies: Introducing clean cooking solutions, such as improved cookstoves and renewable energy alternatives, reduces indoor and outdoor PM2.5 pollution in rural areas.

- Sustainable Agriculture Practices: Implementing precision farming, organic agriculture, and sustainable land management practices minimizes the release of particulate matter from agricultural activities.

- Community Engagement: Fostering community-led initiatives, promoting education on air quality, and empowering rural populations to adopt sustainable practices contribute to building resilience against PM2.5 pollution.

Integrated Approaches:

- Regional Collaboration: Recognizing the interdependence of urban and rural areas, regional collaboration is essential. Shared strategies, data exchange, and coordinated efforts contribute to holistic air quality management.

- Policy Frameworks: Governments play a pivotal role in formulating and enforcing policies that address PM2.5 pollution. Stringent emission standards, incentive programs, and regulatory frameworks contribute to creating a conducive environment for cleaner practices in both urban and rural settings.

Conclusion: Balancing Progress and Environmental Health

As we unveil the dual face of PM2.5's impact on urban and rural areas, a complex narrative emerges—one that intertwines progress and environmental health. The challenge lies in navigating this intricate tapestry, balancing the aspirations of urbanization and economic growth with the imperative to safeguard the well-being of diverse communities.

In the chapters that follow, we will delve into specific case studies, success stories, and ongoing challenges in both urban and rural landscapes, aiming to unravel the complexities of managing PM2.5 pollution on a localized scale. The journey toward cleaner air involves not only understanding the distinct challenges faced by urban and rural areas but also fostering a collective commitment to creating environments where progress harmonizes with environmental health.

Consequences for Developing and Developed Nations

The impact of PM2.5 pollution reverberates across the global landscape, but its consequences unfold with distinct nuances in developing and developed nations. This chapter explores how fine particulate matter shapes the trajectories of progress and environmental health, shedding light on the disparities and common challenges faced by nations at different stages of development.

Developing Nations: The Struggle for Balance

In developing nations, where economic growth often takes precedence over environmental considerations, the consequences of PM2.5 pollution manifest in ways that underscore the delicate balance between development and environmental health.

Industrialization and Air Quality: The rapid industrialization characteristic of many developing nations contributes significantly to elevated levels of PM2.5. As industries burgeon to meet growing demands, emissions from manufacturing processes, energy production, and the use of outdated technologies become major sources of fine particulate matter. The pursuit of economic development, while crucial for lifting populations out of poverty, often collides with the imperative to safeguard air quality.

Urbanization Challenges: Developing nations experience accelerated urbanization as rural populations migrate to cities in search of economic opportunities. The resultant increase in vehicular traffic, energy consumption, and industrial activities amplifies PM2.5 pollution in urban centers. Unplanned urbanization, inadequate infrastructure, and a lack of regulatory enforcement further compound the challenges of managing air quality in rapidly growing cities.

Health Disparities: The health impacts of PM2.5 pollution in developing nations disproportionately affect vulnerable populations. Limited access to healthcare, inadequate sanitation, and pre-existing health conditions amplify the risks associated with fine particulate matter exposure. Respiratory diseases, cardiovascular ailments, and adverse pregnancy outcomes become prevalent health concerns, creating a public health crisis that demands urgent attention.

Economic Implications: Developing nations grapple with the economic repercussions of PM2.5 pollution, affecting both productivity and healthcare expenditures. The costs of treating air pollution-related diseases, combined with productivity losses due to illness and premature mortality, create a considerable economic burden. Striking a balance between economic growth and environmental sustainability becomes a central challenge for policymakers in developing nations.

Socioeconomic Disparities: Within the context of developing nations, socioeconomic disparities exacerbate the impact of PM2.5 pollution. Marginalized communities often bear a disproportionate burden of exposure, residing in close proximity to industrial zones and facing inadequate access to clean resources. Environmental justice becomes a critical consideration as policymakers strive to address the unequal distribution of the health impacts of PM2.5 pollution.

Technological Transition Challenges: Developing nations face challenges in transitioning to cleaner technologies due to economic constraints and a reliance on traditional, pollutant-emitting practices. The need for sustainable development becomes a central theme, requiring a careful balancing act to harness economic growth while mitigating the environmental impact of PM2.5 pollution.

Developed Nations: Navigating the Complexities of Progress

In contrast, developed nations, while often boasting cleaner air quality compared to their developing counterparts, face their own set of challenges and consequences associated with PM2.5 pollution.

Technological Advancements and Emission Control: Developed nations leverage technological advancements and stringent environmental regulations to control and reduce emissions of fine particulate matter. Industries adopt cleaner technologies, emission control devices, and sustainable practices, contributing to overall improvements in air quality. The implementation of strict emission standards and regulatory frameworks becomes a cornerstone of air quality management.

Urban Planning and Sustainable Practices: Developed nations prioritize sustainable urban planning, emphasizing public transportation, green spaces, and emission reduction initiatives. Well-designed cities, stringent building codes, and effective waste management contribute to lower levels of PM2.5

pollution in urban centers. The focus on sustainability aligns with broader environmental goals and enhances the quality of life for urban populations.

Health Monitoring and Access to Healthcare: The emphasis on healthcare infrastructure and monitoring systems allows developed nations to track and address the health impacts of PM2.5 pollution more effectively. Accessible healthcare services, public awareness campaigns, and research initiatives contribute to mitigating the health consequences associated with fine particulate matter exposure.

Economic Resilience: Developed nations exhibit economic resilience in the face of PM2.5 pollution, with robust healthcare systems and productivity gains resulting from improved air quality. The economic costs associated with air pollution-related illnesses are comparatively lower, allowing for investments in sustainable technologies and clean energy initiatives.

International Collaboration: Developed nations often play a key role in international collaborations and initiatives aimed at addressing global air quality challenges. Sharing best practices, technological innovations, and financial resources fosters a collaborative approach to tackling the transboundary impacts of PM2.5 pollution.

Environmental Stewardship and Climate Goals: Environmental stewardship and adherence to climate goals become integral components of the policies of developed nations. The recognition of the interconnectedness between air quality, climate change, and human health shapes strategies that align with international agreements and contribute to the broader goal of sustainable development.

Common Challenges and Shared Responsibilities

While the consequences of PM2.5 pollution differ between developing and developed nations, there are common challenges that underscore the shared responsibility of the global community in addressing this pervasive issue.

Climate Change Interactions: PM2.5 pollution interacts with broader climate change dynamics, influencing weather patterns, and precipitation. Both developing and developed nations grapple with the consequences of changing climates, emphasizing the need for coordinated efforts to address the interlinked challenges of air quality and climate change.

Global Economic Costs: The economic costs associated with PM2.5 pollution extend beyond national borders. Healthcare expenditures, productivity losses, and the broader socio-economic impacts demand a global commitment to mitigating the financial toll of air pollution. Collaborative initiatives, financial support for developing nations, and technology transfer become essential components of global strategies.

Technology Transfer and Capacity Building: Bridging the technological gap between developed and developing nations requires concerted efforts in technology transfer and capacity building. Developed nations can play a pivotal role in supporting the adoption of cleaner technologies, providing expertise, and enhancing the capacity of developing nations to address PM2.5 pollution effectively.

International Cooperation: The consequences of PM2.5 pollution underscore the interconnectedness of nations and the shared responsibility in safeguarding global air quality. International cooperation, multilateral agreements, and collaborative frameworks become indispensable tools in addressing the transboundary impacts of fine particulate matter.

Inclusive Policy Frameworks: Developing inclusive policy frameworks that account for the unique challenges of both developing and developed nations is crucial. Policies should prioritize sustainable development, equitable distribution of environmental resources, and strategies that balance economic growth with environmental health.

Moving Forward: A Global Commitment to Clean Air

As the global community grapples with the consequences of PM2.5 pollution, the path forward necessitates a collective commitment to clean air that transcends national boundaries. Bridging the disparities between developing and developed nations requires a nuanced understanding of the challenges, shared responsibilities, and the recognition that the quest for clean air is an integral aspect of sustainable development.

In the chapters that follow, we will delve into specific case studies, success stories, and ongoing challenges in both developing and developed nations, aiming to unravel the complexities of managing PM2.5 pollution on a global scale. The journey toward cleaner air involves not only acknowledging the disparities in impacts but also fostering a collective commitment to creating a global environment where progress harmonizes with environmental health.

Chapter 3: Health Impacts

Respiratory Health Issues

As the global prevalence of PM2.5 pollution continues to rise, its profound impact on respiratory health emerges as a central concern. This chapter delves into the intricate relationship between fine particulate matter and respiratory health, unraveling the spectrum of consequences that individuals face when exposed to elevated levels of PM2.5.

Understanding the Respiratory System: A Complex Web of Functionality

The respiratory system, comprising the airways, lungs, and associated structures, plays a vital role in supplying oxygen to the body and expelling carbon dioxide. Fine particulate matter, with its microscopic size, poses a unique threat to the delicate balance within the respiratory system.

Airway Entrapment and Alveolar Penetration: PM2.5 particles, being exceptionally small, can penetrate deep into the respiratory system. While larger particles may be trapped in the nose and upper airways, PM2.5 can reach the lower airways and alveoli. The deposition of these particles triggers a cascade of physiological responses, setting the stage for respiratory health issues.

Inflammatory Responses: When PM2.5 particles reach the lungs, they activate inflammatory responses as the body attempts to clear the foreign invaders. This inflammatory process involves the release of cytokines, recruitment of immune cells, and the initiation of oxidative stress. Prolonged exposure to PM2.5 can result in chronic inflammation, contributing to the development of respiratory conditions.

Oxidative Stress and Cellular Damage: The small size of PM2.5 allows it to carry reactive components, leading to oxidative stress within lung cells. Oxidative stress, characterized by an imbalance between antioxidants and reactive oxygen species, can damage cellular structures and DNA. Over time, this damage contributes to the progression of respiratory diseases.

Acute Effects of PM2.5 Exposure on the Respiratory System

Short-term exposure to elevated levels of PM2.5 can induce acute effects on the respiratory system, causing discomfort and exacerbating pre-existing conditions.

Aggravation of Respiratory Symptoms: Individuals with pre-existing respiratory conditions, such as asthma or chronic obstructive pulmonary disease (COPD), may experience exacerbated symptoms during periods of high PM2.5 concentrations. Increased coughing, shortness of breath, and chest tightness are common manifestations of acute exposure.

Increased Respiratory Infections: PM2.5 exposure has been linked to an increased susceptibility to respiratory infections, including bronchitis and pneumonia. The compromised immune response in the presence of PM2.5 can facilitate the entry and replication of pathogens, leading to heightened infection risks.

Exacerbation of Allergies: For individuals with respiratory allergies, exposure to PM2.5 can trigger or worsen allergic reactions. The inflammatory responses induced by fine particulate matter can amplify the body's sensitivity to allergens, contributing to the exacerbation of allergic respiratory conditions.

Cardio-Respiratory Interactions: The effects of PM2.5 on the respiratory system are interconnected with cardiovascular consequences. Short-term exposure can lead to increased heart rate, changes in blood pressure, and vascular dysfunction. These interactions highlight the holistic impact of PM2.5 on the cardio-respiratory system.

Long-term Consequences: Chronic Respiratory Diseases and Beyond

The chronic exposure to elevated levels of PM2.5 is associated with the development and progression of various respiratory diseases, presenting long-term challenges to public health.

Chronic Obstructive Pulmonary Disease (COPD): Long-term exposure to PM2.5 is a recognized risk factor for the development and exacerbation of COPD. The chronic inflammation and oxidative stress induced by fine particulate matter contribute to the progressive damage of airways and lung tissue, leading to persistent airflow limitation.

**Asthma: ** Individuals with asthma face an increased risk of asthma exacerbations and impaired asthma control in the presence of elevated PM2.5 levels. Fine particulate matter can trigger bronchoconstriction, airway inflammation, and heightened respiratory symptoms in asthmatic individuals.

Interstitial Lung Diseases: Chronic exposure to PM2.5 has been linked to the development of interstitial lung diseases, characterized by inflammation and scarring of the lung tissue. These conditions, including idiopathic pulmonary fibrosis, pose significant challenges for affected individuals, as the lung's ability to exchange oxygen becomes compromised.

Lung Cancer: While the primary risk factor for lung cancer is tobacco smoke, there is evidence linking long-term exposure to PM2.5 with an increased risk of lung cancer. Fine particulate matter carries carcinogenic components and contributes to the formation of DNA-damaging reactive oxygen species, creating a conducive environment for the initiation and progression of cancerous cells.

Reduced Lung Function and Growth: Children exposed to elevated levels of PM2.5 may experience impaired lung development and reduced lung function. The impact of fine particulate matter on respiratory health during critical developmental stages can have lasting consequences, affecting lung growth and function throughout life.

Vulnerable Populations: Understanding Disparities in Respiratory Health Impacts

Certain populations are more vulnerable to the respiratory health impacts of PM2.5 pollution, emphasizing the need for targeted interventions and protective measures.

Children: Developing respiratory systems make children more susceptible to the effects of PM2.5. Long-term exposure can lead to reduced lung growth, increased respiratory infections, and heightened risks of asthma development.

Childhood exposure to fine particulate matter sets the stage for a lifetime of respiratory health challenges.

Elderly Individuals: Aging is associated with a natural decline in lung function, making elderly individuals more susceptible to the adverse effects of PM2.5. Chronic exposure can exacerbate age-related respiratory conditions and contribute to an increased burden of respiratory diseases among the elderly.

Individuals with Pre-existing Conditions: Those with pre-existing respiratory conditions, such as asthma, COPD, or cardiovascular diseases, face amplified risks from PM2.5 exposure. The inflammatory responses triggered by fine particulate matter can further compromise the respiratory and cardiovascular systems in individuals already grappling with chronic health issues.

Low Socioeconomic Status: Individuals with lower socioeconomic status often face higher levels of PM2.5 exposure due to living in areas with inadequate air quality, limited access to healthcare, and proximity to industrial zones. Socioeconomic disparities contribute to an unequal distribution of respiratory health impacts, underscoring the importance of addressing environmental justice in air quality management.

Mitigation Strategies: Safeguarding Respiratory Health in a PM2.5-Prone World

Addressing the respiratory health impacts of PM2.5 pollution requires a comprehensive approach encompassing public health interventions, regulatory measures, and technological advancements.

Air Quality Monitoring and Alerts: Implementing robust air quality monitoring systems allows for timely alerts and public notifications during periods of elevated PM2.5 concentrations. Providing real-time information empowers individuals to take preventive measures, especially vulnerable populations.

Regulatory Measures: Stringent regulations and emission standards play a crucial role in controlling sources of PM2.5 pollution. Implementing and enforcing measures to limit industrial emissions, vehicle exhaust, and other anthropogenic sources contribute to reducing ambient concentrations.

Green Spaces and Urban Planning: Incorporating green spaces, urban forests, and sustainable urban planning practices enhances air quality in urban environments. Vegetation serves as a natural filter, absorbing particulate matter and contributing to a healthier urban atmosphere.

Public Awareness and Education: Raising public awareness about the respiratory health impacts of PM2.5 is essential for fostering behavioral changes and encouraging individuals to take protective measures. Education campaigns, community workshops, and school programs contribute to building a knowledgeable and empowered populace.

Technological Innovations: Advancements in clean technologies, including electric vehicles, renewable energy sources, and emission control devices, play a pivotal role in reducing the anthropogenic sources of PM2.5 pollution.

Supporting and incentivizing the adoption of cleaner technologies contribute to overall air quality improvement.

Healthcare Interventions: Accessible healthcare services, particularly for vulnerable populations, are critical for managing respiratory health issues associated with PM2.5 exposure. Early diagnosis, treatment, and ongoing care contribute to mitigating the impacts of respiratory diseases.

International Cooperation: Given the transboundary nature of air pollution, international collaboration is essential in addressing the global respiratory health impacts of PM2.5. Sharing best practices, collaborative research initiatives, and supporting developing nations in air quality management contribute to a concerted global effort.

Conclusion: Navigating the Breath of Consequences

As we navigate the intricate web of consequences stemming from PM2.5 exposure on respiratory health, a nuanced understanding of the challenges and potential solutions emerges. The journey toward safeguarding respiratory health in a PM2.5-prone world involves not only addressing the acute and chronic impacts on individuals but also fostering a collective commitment to creating environments where every breath is a testament to clean air and well-being.

In the chapters that follow, we will delve into specific case studies, success stories, and ongoing challenges related to respiratory health impacts, aiming to unravel the complexities of managing PM2.5 pollution on a global scale. The journey toward cleaner air involves not only acknowledging the breadth of consequences but also fostering a collective commitment to creating a world where respiratory health is prioritized and protected.

Cardiovascular Effects

As PM2.5 pollution permeates the global atmosphere, its impact extends beyond the respiratory system, casting a shadow over cardiovascular health. This chapter unravels the intricate relationship between fine particulate matter and cardiovascular effects, exploring the multifaceted consequences that arise when individuals are exposed to elevated levels of PM2.5.

The Cardiovascular System: A Symphony of Functionality

The cardiovascular system, comprising the heart, blood vessels, and associated structures, orchestrates the circulation of blood throughout the body. PM2.5, with its ability to penetrate deep into the lungs and enter the bloodstream, sets the stage for a range of cardiovascular effects.

Systemic Circulation: Once inhaled, PM2.5 particles can bypass the respiratory defenses and enter the bloodstream directly. This allows the particles to be transported to various organs and tissues, exerting systemic effects on the cardiovascular system.

Inflammatory Responses: The presence of PM2.5 in the bloodstream triggers inflammatory responses, involving the release of cytokines and activation of immune cells. Chronic inflammation, induced by persistent exposure to fine particulate matter, contributes to the development and progression of cardiovascular diseases.

Oxidative Stress: PM2.5 particles carry reactive components that can lead to oxidative stress within blood vessels and the heart. The imbalance between antioxidants and reactive oxygen species promotes cellular damage, lipid peroxidation, and vascular dysfunction, laying the groundwork for cardiovascular issues.

Acute Cardiovascular Effects: Unraveling the Immediate Impact

Short-term exposure to elevated levels of PM2.5 is associated with acute cardiovascular effects, manifesting in changes to heart rate, blood pressure, and vascular function.

Increased Heart Rate: Fine particulate matter can lead to an increase in heart rate as the body responds to the presence of PM2.5 in the bloodstream. This acute physiological response is part of the cardiovascular system's attempt to cope with the stress imposed by exposure to fine particulate matter.

Changes in Blood Pressure: PM2.5 exposure has been linked to both increases in systolic and diastolic blood pressure. Elevated blood pressure levels contribute to the strain on the cardiovascular system, increasing the risk of hypertension and related complications.

Vascular Dysfunction: The presence of PM2.5 can impair the function of blood vessels, leading to endothelial dysfunction. Endothelial cells, lining the interior of blood vessels, play a crucial role in regulating vascular tone and maintaining blood flow. Dysfunction in these cells contributes to the development of cardiovascular diseases.

Arrhythmias: Acute exposure to PM2.5 has been associated with an increased risk of arrhythmias, irregular heartbeats that can have serious implications for cardiovascular health. The mechanisms underlying these arrhythmias involve the disruption of electrical signaling within the heart.

Long-term Consequences: Chronic Cardiovascular Diseases

The chronic exposure to elevated levels of PM2.5 poses significant risks for the development and progression of various cardiovascular diseases, contributing to a global burden of morbidity and mortality.

Hypertension: Chronic exposure to PM2.5 is a recognized risk factor for the development of hypertension, a condition characterized by sustained high blood pressure. Hypertension, when left uncontrolled, increases the risk of heart disease, stroke, and other cardiovascular complications.

Atherosclerosis: PM2.5 has been linked to the development of atherosclerosis, a condition characterized by the buildup of plaque within arteries. The inflammatory and oxidative stress responses induced by fine particulate matter contribute to the progression of atherosclerotic lesions, narrowing blood vessels and impeding blood flow.

Coronary Artery Disease: The association between chronic PM2.5 exposure and the development of coronary artery disease underscores the role of fine particulate matter in compromising the blood supply to the heart. Coronary artery disease, marked by the narrowing of coronary arteries, poses a significant risk of heart attacks and heart-related complications.

Heart Failure: Prolonged exposure to PM2.5 is associated with an increased risk of heart failure, a condition in which the heart is unable to pump blood efficiently. The inflammatory and oxidative stress responses induced by fine particulate matter contribute to the structural and functional changes in the heart that underlie heart failure.

Stroke: The cardiovascular consequences of PM2.5 extend to an increased risk of stroke. The systemic effects of fine particulate matter, including inflammation, oxidative stress, and vascular dysfunction, create an environment conducive to the development of cerebrovascular diseases.

Cardiovascular Mortality: Chronic exposure to elevated levels of PM2.5 is a significant contributor to cardiovascular mortality. The increased risk of heart attacks, strokes, and other cardiovascular events underscores the life-threatening impact of fine particulate matter on the global population.

Vulnerable Populations: Disparities in Cardiovascular Health Impacts

Certain populations are more vulnerable to the cardiovascular effects of PM2.5 pollution, emphasizing the need for targeted interventions and protective measures.

Elderly Individuals: Aging is associated with a natural decline in cardiovascular function, making elderly individuals more susceptible to the cardiovascular effects of PM2.5. Chronic exposure can exacerbate age-related cardiovascular conditions, contributing to an increased burden of cardiovascular diseases among the elderly.

Individuals with Pre-existing Cardiovascular Conditions: Those with pre-existing cardiovascular conditions, such as hypertension, coronary artery disease, or heart failure, face amplified risks from PM2.5 exposure. The inflammatory and oxidative stress responses induced by fine particulate matter can further compromise the cardiovascular system in individuals already grappling with chronic health issues.

Diabetic Individuals: Diabetes is a known risk factor for cardiovascular diseases, and individuals with diabetes may face heightened susceptibility to the cardiovascular effects of PM2.5. The interactions between PM2.5-induced inflammation and oxidative stress and the underlying mechanisms of diabetes contribute to an increased risk of cardiovascular complications.

Low Socioeconomic Status: Individuals with lower socioeconomic status often face higher levels of PM2.5 exposure due to living in areas with inadequate air quality, limited access to healthcare, and proximity to industrial zones. Socioeconomic disparities contribute to an unequal distribution of cardiovascular health impacts, underscoring the importance of addressing environmental justice in air quality management.

Mitigation Strategies: Safeguarding Cardiovascular Health in a PM2.5-Prone World

Addressing the cardiovascular effects of PM2.5 pollution necessitates a comprehensive approach that encompasses public health interventions, regulatory measures, and technological advancements.

Air Quality Standards and Regulations: Establishing and enforcing stringent air quality standards and regulations is fundamental to controlling and reducing PM2.5 pollution. Emission controls, industrial regulations, and vehicle standards contribute to mitigating the sources of fine particulate matter.

Public Health Interventions: Public awareness campaigns, targeted at informing individuals about the cardiovascular effects of PM2.5, play a crucial role in fostering behavioral changes. Public health initiatives can include educational programs, community outreach, and interventions aimed at vulnerable populations.

Green Spaces and Urban Planning: Incorporating green spaces, parks, and urban planning practices that prioritize cardiovascular health contributes to a healthier urban environment. Access to green spaces has been associated with reduced cardiovascular risks, providing a natural countermeasure to the effects of PM2.5.

Technological Innovations: Advancements in clean technologies, including electric vehicles, renewable energy sources, and emission control devices, contribute to reducing anthropogenic sources of PM2.5 pollution. Supporting and incentivizing the adoption of cleaner technologies play a pivotal role in improving air quality and cardiovascular health.

Cardiovascular Health Monitoring: Implementing robust cardiovascular health monitoring systems allows for the early detection and management of cardiovascular issues associated with PM2.5 exposure. Regular health check-ups, especially for vulnerable populations, contribute to timely interventions and improved outcomes.

International Collaboration: Given the global nature of air pollution, international collaboration is essential in addressing the cardiovascular health impacts of PM2.5. Sharing best practices, collaborative research initiatives, and supporting developing nations in air quality management contribute to a concerted global effort.

Conclusion: The Heart of the Matter

As we navigate the pervasive influence of PM2.5 on cardiovascular health, a comprehensive understanding of the intricate web of consequences emerges. The journey toward safeguarding cardiovascular health in a PM2.5-prone world involves not only unraveling the immediate and chronic impacts on individuals but also fostering a collective commitment to creating environments where every heartbeat resonates with the rhythm of clean air and well-being.

In the chapters that follow, we will delve into specific case studies, success stories, and ongoing challenges related to cardiovascular health impacts, aiming to unravel the complexities of managing PM2.5 pollution on a global scale. The journey toward cleaner air involves not only acknowledging the breadth of consequences but also fostering a collective commitment to creating a world where cardiovascular health is prioritized and protected.

Long-term Health Consequences

As PM2.5 pollution persists in our global atmosphere, the implications for long-term health consequences become increasingly evident. This chapter explores the enduring impact of fine particulate matter on human health, delving into the complex web of consequences that unfold over time.

Chronic Exposure Dynamics: Unraveling the Cumulative Effects

Chronic exposure to elevated levels of PM2.5 sets the stage for a myriad of long-term health consequences, influencing various organ systems and contributing to the burden of chronic diseases.

Systemic Inflammation: One of the hallmark features of long-term PM2.5 exposure is the induction of systemic inflammation. Fine particulate matter, once inhaled, initiates a cascade of inflammatory responses throughout the body. Persistent inflammation becomes a driving force behind the development and progression of chronic diseases.

Oxidative Stress: The oxidative stress induced by PM2.5, characterized by an imbalance between reactive oxygen species and antioxidants, becomes a pervasive feature of chronic exposure. Over time, this oxidative burden contributes to cellular damage, DNA mutations, and the gradual deterioration of physiological functions.

Epigenetic Changes: Long-term exposure to PM2.5 has been associated with epigenetic modifications, altering gene expression patterns without changes to the underlying DNA sequence. These changes can influence susceptibility to various diseases and contribute to the heritability of health impacts across generations.

Organ-Specific Effects: Different organs exhibit distinct responses to chronic PM2.5 exposure. The lungs, heart, brain, liver, and other vital organs may undergo structural and functional changes, leading to a spectrum of health issues.

Respiratory System: A Persistent Battleground

The respiratory system bears the brunt of long-term PM2.5 exposure, experiencing a cascade of consequences that unfold over the years.

Chronic Obstructive Pulmonary Disease (COPD): Long-term exposure to fine particulate matter is a significant risk factor for the development and progression of COPD. The chronic inflammation and oxidative stress induced by PM2.5 contribute to the progressive damage of airways and lung tissue, leading to persistent airflow limitation.

Asthma Exacerbation and Persistence: Individuals with asthma face ongoing challenges in managing their condition under the persistent influence of PM2.5. Long-term exposure is associated with increased asthma exacerbations, worsened symptoms, and the potential for the persistence of respiratory issues.

Interstitial Lung Diseases: Chronic exposure to PM2.5 has been linked to the development of interstitial lung diseases, characterized by inflammation and scarring of the lung tissue. These conditions, including idiopathic pulmonary fibrosis, pose significant challenges for affected individuals, as the lung's ability to exchange oxygen becomes compromised.

Lung Cancer Risk: While tobacco smoke remains the primary risk factor for lung cancer, long-term exposure to PM2.5 has been identified as a contributing factor. Fine particulate matter carries carcinogenic components and contributes to the formation of DNA-damaging reactive oxygen species, creating conditions conducive to the initiation and progression of lung cancer.

Cardiovascular System: The Unrelenting Toll

The cardiovascular system, intimately linked to respiratory health, bears the enduring burden of PM2.5 exposure, contributing to a spectrum of chronic cardiovascular diseases.

Hypertension and Vascular Dysfunction: Long-term exposure to PM2.5 is a recognized risk factor for the development of hypertension. The inflammatory responses, oxidative stress, and endothelial dysfunction induced by fine particulate matter contribute to sustained high blood pressure, increasing the risk of cardiovascular complications.

Atherosclerosis and Coronary Artery Disease: Chronic exposure to PM2.5 is implicated in the progression of atherosclerosis and the development of coronary artery disease. The systemic effects of fine particulate matter contribute to the buildup of plaque within arteries, narrowing blood vessels and impeding blood flow to the heart.

Arrhythmias and Heart Failure: The chronic cardiovascular effects of PM2.5 extend to an increased risk of arrhythmias and heart failure. Persistent exposure disrupts the electrical signaling within the heart and contributes to structural changes that underlie these cardiovascular conditions.

Stroke and Cerebrovascular Diseases: Long-term exposure to elevated levels of PM2.5 is associated with an increased risk of stroke. The systemic impact of fine particulate matter creates an environment conducive to the development of cerebrovascular diseases, further contributing to the burden of cardiovascular morbidity.

Neurological Impact: Unraveling the Mind-Body Connection

Emerging evidence suggests that long-term exposure to PM2.5 can influence neurological health, with implications for cognitive function and the risk of neurodegenerative diseases.

Neuroinflammation and Cognitive Decline: Chronic exposure to fine particulate matter has been linked to neuroinflammation, contributing to the gradual decline in cognitive function. Long-term consequences may include an increased risk of neurodegenerative diseases such as Alzheimer's and Parkinson's.

Impact on Mental Health: The systemic effects of PM2.5 can extend to mental health, with chronic exposure being associated with an increased risk of conditions such as depression and anxiety. The inflammatory and oxidative stress responses induced by fine particulate matter may contribute to alterations in neurotransmitter function and neuronal signaling.

Reproductive and Developmental Consequences: A Generational Echo

The enduring impact of PM2.5 exposure extends to reproductive health, influencing fertility, pregnancy outcomes, and the long-term health of the next generation.

Fertility Issues: Long-term exposure to PM2.5 has been linked to fertility issues in both men and women. The impact on reproductive health may include reduced fertility, impaired sperm quality, and disruptions to hormonal balance.

Pregnancy Complications: Pregnant individuals exposed to elevated levels of PM2.5 face an increased risk of complications, including preterm birth, low birth weight, and developmental issues. The systemic effects of fine particulate matter may influence placental function and fetal development.

Early Life Exposures and Lifelong Impact: Exposures to elevated levels of PM2.5 during early life stages can have lifelong consequences. Children born to mothers exposed to PM2.5 may face heightened risks of respiratory issues, developmental challenges, and an increased susceptibility to chronic diseases later in life.

Beyond Physical Health: Societal and Economic Impact

The long-term health consequences of PM2.5 pollution extend beyond individual well-being, impacting societal health, economic productivity, and the overall quality of life.

Healthcare Burden: The chronic diseases resulting from long-term PM2.5 exposure contribute significantly to the healthcare burden. The increased prevalence of respiratory, cardiovascular, and neurological conditions places strain on healthcare systems and resources.

Productivity Loss: Individuals grappling with chronic health conditions may experience reduced productivity, affecting economic output at both individual and societal levels. The economic impact of PM2.5-induced health consequences extends to absenteeism, disability, and increased healthcare costs.

Health Disparities: Vulnerable populations, often disproportionately exposed to higher levels of PM2.5, bear a greater burden of long-term health consequences. Socioeconomic disparities contribute to disparities in health outcomes, creating an urgent need for equitable interventions and environmental justice.

Mitigation Strategies: Navigating Towards a Healthier Future

Mitigating the long-term health consequences of PM2.5 exposure requires a multifaceted approach encompassing public health interventions, regulatory measures, technological innovations, and global collaboration.

Emission Controls and Air Quality Standards: Stringent emission controls and air quality standards are fundamental in reducing and controlling the sources of PM2.5 pollution. Regulatory measures aimed at industries, transportation, and other anthropogenic sources contribute to creating a healthier ambient air environment.

Public Health Education: Raising awareness about the long-term health consequences of PM2.5 is crucial for fostering individual and collective actions. Public health education campaigns, school programs, and community engagement initiatives play a vital role in disseminating knowledge and encouraging behavioral changes.

Green Infrastructure and Urban Planning: Incorporating green infrastructure, urban forests, and sustainable urban planning practices contribute to reducing ambient concentrations of PM2.5. Green spaces act as natural filters, enhancing air quality and promoting overall well-being.

International Cooperation: Addressing the global challenge of long-term health consequences from PM2.5 pollution requires international collaboration. Sharing best practices, supporting developing nations in air quality management, and advancing joint research initiatives contribute to a concerted global effort.

Technological Innovations: Advancements in clean technologies, such as electric vehicles, renewable energy sources, and efficient industrial processes, contribute to reducing anthropogenic sources of PM2.5. Investing in and incentivizing the adoption of cleaner technologies play a pivotal role in improving air quality and mitigating long-term health consequences.

Environmental Justice: Prioritizing environmental justice is essential in addressing health disparities associated with long-term PM2.5 exposure. Equitable distribution of resources, access to healthcare, and targeted interventions for vulnerable populations contribute to creating a more just and inclusive approach to air quality management.

Conclusion: Navigating the Endurance

As we navigate the enduring impact of PM2.5 on human health, a comprehensive understanding of the long-term consequences emerges. The journey toward mitigating these consequences involves not only unraveling the intricate web of health effects but also fostering a collective commitment to creating environments where health endures and thrives.

In the chapters that follow, we will delve into specific case studies, success stories, and ongoing challenges related to long-term health consequences, aiming to unravel the complexities of managing PM2.5 pollution on a global scale. The journey towards cleaner air involves not only acknowledging the enduring consequences but also fostering a collective commitment to creating a world where health stands resilient against the enduring influence of fine particulate matter.

Vulnerable Populations and Demographic Variances

As the global challenge of PM2.5 pollution unfolds, it becomes evident that certain populations are more vulnerable to its health impacts. This chapter explores the intricate landscape of vulnerability, shedding light on demographic variances and the disparities that shape the health outcomes of those exposed to elevated levels of fine particulate matter.

Understanding Vulnerability: A Multifaceted Lens

Vulnerability to the health impacts of PM2.5 is influenced by a complex interplay of factors, encompassing demographic, socioeconomic, environmental, and health-related elements. Certain populations face heightened susceptibility, emphasizing the need for targeted interventions and a nuanced understanding of vulnerability.

Demographic Variances: A Mosaic of Vulnerability

Children and Adolescents: The developing bodies and immune systems of children make them particularly susceptible to the health impacts of PM2.5. Long-term exposure during critical developmental stages can result in respiratory issues, impaired lung growth, and increased vulnerability to infections.

Elderly Individuals: Aging is associated with a natural decline in physiological resilience, rendering elderly individuals more susceptible to the health effects of PM2.5. Pre-existing health conditions, decreased lung function, and compromised immune responses contribute to heightened vulnerability.

Individuals with Pre-existing Health Conditions: Those already grappling with chronic health conditions, such as respiratory diseases, cardiovascular issues, or diabetes, face amplified risks from PM2.5 exposure. The interaction between fine particulate matter and pre-existing health conditions exacerbates the severity of health outcomes.

Pregnant Individuals: Pregnancy introduces unique vulnerabilities, as the developing fetus is intricately connected to the health of the mother. PM2.5 exposure during pregnancy is associated with adverse outcomes, including preterm birth, low birth weight, and developmental issues.

Socioeconomic Disparities: Vulnerability to PM2.5 health impacts is often intertwined with socioeconomic factors. Individuals in lower socioeconomic strata may face higher exposure levels due to residence in areas with poor air quality, limited access to healthcare, and proximity to industrial zones.

Health Disparities: A Tale of Inequitable Burdens

Respiratory Health Disparities: Vulnerable populations, including children and individuals with lower socioeconomic status, often bear a disproportionate burden of respiratory health impacts. Asthma exacerbations, chronic bronchitis, and other respiratory conditions showcase the stark health disparities associated with PM2.5 exposure.

Cardiovascular Health Disparities: The cardiovascular effects of PM2.5 contribute to disparities in cardiovascular health outcomes. Vulnerable populations, such as the elderly and those with pre-existing cardiovascular conditions, face an increased risk of hypertension, atherosclerosis, and other cardiovascular issues.

Reproductive and Developmental Health Disparities: Vulnerable populations, particularly pregnant individuals with limited access to healthcare, may experience heightened risks during pregnancy. Adverse outcomes, such as preterm birth and low birth weight, underscore the importance of addressing reproductive and developmental health disparities.

Geographical Disparities: The uneven distribution of PM2.5 pollution contributes to geographical disparities in health impacts. Urban areas with high traffic density, industrial zones, and limited green spaces may harbor elevated levels of fine particulate matter, impacting the health of residents.

Occupational Exposures: Certain occupations expose individuals to higher levels of PM2.5, leading to occupational health disparities. Workers in industries such as construction, manufacturing, and transportation face increased risks, emphasizing the need for workplace regulations and protective measures.

Access to Healthcare: Disparities in access to healthcare compound the challenges faced by vulnerable populations. Limited access to medical services, preventive care, and timely interventions may exacerbate the health impacts of PM2.5, creating an urgent need for healthcare equity.

Environmental Justice: Vulnerable populations often reside in areas with inadequate environmental protection and limited resources. Environmental justice considerations highlight the importance of equitable distribution of resources, fair access to clean air, and inclusive decision-making in air quality management.

Navigating Vulnerability: Tailoring Interventions for Impact

Early Childhood Interventions: Targeting interventions during early childhood is crucial for mitigating the long-term health impacts of PM2.5. Educational programs, community initiatives, and policy measures focused on reducing childhood exposure contribute to building a healthier future.

Elderly Care and Support: Providing specialized care and support for the elderly population helps address the unique vulnerabilities associated with aging. Healthcare services, community programs, and public health campaigns tailored to the needs of elderly individuals contribute to enhanced resilience.

Preventive Healthcare for High-Risk Groups: Individuals with pre-existing health conditions benefit from targeted preventive healthcare. Regular health check-ups, disease management programs, and public health campaigns aimed at high-risk groups contribute to early detection and intervention.

Prenatal and Maternal Healthcare: Ensuring access to quality prenatal and maternal healthcare is pivotal for mitigating the reproductive and developmental health impacts of PM2.5. Integrated healthcare services, education, and support for pregnant individuals contribute to positive outcomes.

Socioeconomic Support Programs: Addressing socioeconomic disparities requires comprehensive support programs. Accessible healthcare services, educational initiatives, housing improvements, and employment opportunities contribute to reducing vulnerability in lower socioeconomic strata.

Community Engagement and Empowerment: Empowering communities through engagement initiatives fosters collective resilience. Community-driven projects, environmental education, and advocacy contribute to creating informed and empowered populations capable of advocating for clean air.

Green Infrastructure in Vulnerable Areas: Implementing green infrastructure and urban planning in vulnerable areas enhances the natural filtration of PM2.5. Green spaces, tree planting initiatives, and sustainable urban development contribute to creating healthier living environments.

Environmental Justice Advocacy: Advocacy for environmental justice plays a crucial role in addressing disparities. Engaging in policy discussions, supporting grassroots movements, and advocating for equitable air quality regulations contribute to fostering justice in environmental decision-making.

Global Collaboration for Equitable Solutions: Addressing vulnerability on a global scale requires international collaboration. Sharing best practices, supporting developing nations in air quality management, and advancing joint research initiatives contribute to a concerted global effort.

Conclusion: Navigating Disparities

As we navigate the intricate landscape of vulnerability and disparities associated with PM2.5 exposure, a profound understanding of the multifaceted challenges emerges. The journey toward mitigating health impacts involves not only acknowledging the diverse vulnerabilities but also fostering a collective commitment to creating environments where every individual, regardless of demographic variances, can breathe easy and thrive.

In the chapters that follow, we will delve into specific case studies, success stories, and ongoing challenges related to vulnerable populations and demographic variances, aiming to unravel the complexities of managing PM2.5 pollution on a global scale. The journey towards cleaner air involves not only acknowledging vulnerabilities but also fostering a collective commitment to creating a world where health disparities are addressed and every breath is a testament to equitable well-being.

Chapter 4: Environmental Consequences

Ecosystem Impact

As PM2.5 pollution pervades the atmosphere, its consequences extend beyond human health, casting a looming shadow over ecosystems. This chapter delves into the intricate web of ecosystem impacts, exploring how fine particulate matter disrupts the delicate balance of nature, affecting flora, fauna, and the intricate relationships that sustain our planet.

The Pulse of Ecosystems: Understanding Interconnectedness

Ecosystems, whether terrestrial or aquatic, operate as intricate systems where various components interact in a delicate balance. The introduction of PM2.5 into these ecosystems disrupts this balance, triggering a cascade of consequences that reverberate through the food chain, water bodies, and the very fabric of biodiversity.

Air-Land Interface: Impact on Vegetation

Direct Effects on Plant Physiology: PM2.5, once settled on leaves and surfaces, can directly impact plant physiology. The particles interfere with photosynthesis, reducing the efficiency of light absorption and leading to decreased growth and yield. Stomatal closure, induced by PM2.5, limits gas exchange and nutrient uptake.

Chemical Changes in Soil: The deposition of PM2.5 particles alters soil chemistry. Accumulation of heavy metals, such as lead and cadmium, can occur, posing a threat to plant health. Changes in soil pH and nutrient availability further influence the composition of plant communities.

Changes in Plant Species Composition: Certain plant species prove more resilient to PM2.5 exposure, leading to shifts in plant community composition. This alteration in vegetation dynamics can have cascading effects on herbivores, pollinators, and other organisms dependent on specific plant species.

Aquatic Systems: Impact on Water Bodies

Deposition in Water Bodies: Atmospheric deposition of PM2.5 can result in the introduction of fine particulate matter into water bodies. Rainwater, carrying deposited particles, contributes to the contamination of rivers, lakes, and oceans, impacting aquatic ecosystems.

Water Quality and Aquatic Life: The presence of PM2.5 in water can lead to changes in water quality, affecting the survival and health of aquatic organisms. Fine particulate matter can interfere with nutrient cycling, disrupt aquatic food webs, and contribute to algal blooms, impacting biodiversity.

Bioaccumulation and Biomagnification: PM2.5 particles can be taken up by aquatic organisms. Through processes of bioaccumulation and biomagnification, the concentration of pollutants increases as they move up the food chain. Predatory species at higher trophic levels may face elevated risks of exposure.

Biodiversity Dynamics: Effects on Flora and Fauna

Impact on Wildlife Habitat: Changes in vegetation due to PM2.5 exposure alter wildlife habitats. Animals dependent on specific plant species for food and shelter may face challenges in finding suitable environments, leading to shifts in distribution patterns and potential declines in population.

Disruption of Animal Behavior: Fine particulate matter can interfere with animal behavior. Inhaled particles may impact respiratory systems, alter feeding patterns, or induce stress responses. Behavioral changes in key species can have cascading effects on entire ecosystems.

Population Dynamics: Elevated levels of PM2.5 can influence population dynamics within ecosystems. Changes in reproductive success, survival rates, and migration patterns may occur, affecting the abundance and distribution of species within a given habitat.

Microbial Communities: Unseen Consequences

Soil Microbes and Nutrient Cycling: PM2.5 pollution affects the microbial communities in soil. Soil-dwelling microbes play a crucial role in nutrient cycling, breaking down organic matter and releasing essential nutrients. Changes in microbial composition can disrupt these processes, impacting plant health.

Aquatic Microbes and Water Quality: In aquatic ecosystems, microbial communities contribute to water quality. The introduction of PM2.5 particles can alter the composition and functioning of aquatic microbes, influencing nutrient cycling and the breakdown of organic matter.

Microbial Resilience and Adaptation: Some microbial species may exhibit resilience or adaptation to elevated levels of PM2.5, leading to shifts in microbial community structures.

These changes can have cascading effects on ecosystem processes and the overall health of ecosystems.

Ecosystem Services: A Fragile Balance Disturbed

Impact on Pollination Services: PM2.5 pollution can disrupt pollination services provided by insects, birds, and other pollinators. Reduced flower visitation, altered foraging behavior, and changes in plant-pollinator interactions may compromise the reproduction of flowering plants.

Disruption of Pest Control: Natural predators of pests may be affected by PM2.5 exposure, leading to disruptions in biological pest control mechanisms. Changes in the abundance and behavior of predatory species can result in increased pest populations, affecting crop health.

Water Purification Services: Aquatic ecosystems provide crucial water purification services. PM2.5 pollution in water bodies can compromise these services, impacting the ability of ecosystems to filter contaminants and maintain water quality.

Climate Interactions: A Feedback Loop Unveiled

Contribution to Climate Change: PM2.5 particles can influence climate dynamics. Dark-colored particles, such as black carbon, absorb sunlight, leading to localized warming effects. Changes in the reflective properties of surfaces covered in PM2.5 can contribute to alterations in regional and global climate patterns.

Interaction with Cloud Formation: Fine particulate matter can act as cloud condensation nuclei, influencing cloud formation and properties. This interaction may impact precipitation patterns, affecting the distribution of water resources and contributing to changes in regional climates.

Feedback Loops and Compounded Effects: The interactions between PM2.5 pollution, climate, and ecosystems create complex feedback loops. Climate change influenced by PM2.5 can, in turn, affect ecosystems, leading to compounded and synergistic effects on biodiversity, ecosystem services, and overall environmental health.

Conservation Challenges: Navigating the Ecological Quandary

Loss of Biodiversity: The disruption caused by PM2.5 pollution poses a threat to biodiversity. Habitat alteration, changes in species composition, and population declines may challenge conservation efforts aimed at preserving the richness of ecosystems.

Impacts on Keystone Species: Keystone species, crucial for maintaining ecosystem stability, may be particularly vulnerable to PM2.5 pollution. The loss or decline of keystone species can trigger cascading effects, impacting the structure and function of entire ecosystems.

Resilience and Adaptation Strategies: Ecosystems exhibit varying levels of resilience and adaptation to environmental stressors. Understanding the capacity of ecosystems to recover from PM2.5-induced disruptions is essential for designing effective conservation strategies.

Invasive Species Dynamics: PM2.5 pollution may influence the success and spread of invasive species. Changes in vegetation, disruptions in ecological interactions, and altered resource availability can create conditions conducive to the establishment and dominance of invasive species.

Conservation Policies and Restoration Initiatives: The integration of PM2.5 considerations into conservation policies is crucial. Restoration initiatives focused on improving air quality, reducing pollution sources, and enhancing habitat resilience contribute to the long-term health of ecosystems.

Global Cooperation for Ecosystem Health: Given the transboundary nature of PM2.5 pollution, global cooperation is essential. Collaborative efforts to reduce emissions, protect ecosystems, and address climate change contribute to safeguarding biodiversity on a planetary scale.

Conclusion: Navigating Ecological Consequences

As we navigate the far-reaching consequences of PM2.5 on ecosystems, a profound understanding of the intricate relationships that sustain our planet emerges. The journey toward mitigating ecosystem impacts involves not only unraveling the ecological quandary but also fostering a collective commitment to creating environments where biodiversity thrives, ecosystems flourish, and the delicate balance of nature endures.

In the chapters that follow, we will delve into specific case studies, success stories, and ongoing challenges related to ecosystem impacts, aiming to unravel the complexities of managing PM2.5 pollution on a global scale. The journey towards cleaner air involves not only acknowledging the ecological consequences but also fostering a collective commitment to creating a world where ecosystems are resilient and vibrant against the pervasive influence of fine particulate matter.

Effects on Wildlife

As PM2.5 pollution continues to cast its shadow over the environment, the repercussions extend beyond human health, reaching deep into the realms of wildlife. This chapter delves into the intricate interactions between fine particulate matter and diverse animal species, exploring how the pervasive influence of PM2.5 disrupts ecosystems, alters behavior, and poses challenges to the survival of wildlife.

The Symphony of Nature: Interconnected Lives in the Wild

Wildlife inhabits ecosystems that operate as complex networks of interdependence. From the smallest insects to the largest predators, the impact of PM2.5 pollution weaves through the intricate tapestry of life in the wild, introducing challenges that ripple through entire ecosystems.

Respiratory Challenges: From Avian Highways to Burrows Below

Avian Impacts: Birds, with their high metabolism and efficient respiratory systems, are not exempt from the consequences of PM2.5 exposure. Inhalation of fine particulate matter can lead to respiratory distress, affecting birds both in flight and at rest. Species relying on specialized air sacs for efficient breathing may face heightened vulnerability.

Mammalian Respiratory Health: Terrestrial mammals, ranging from small rodents to large carnivores, can also experience respiratory challenges. PM2.5 inhalation may result in coughing, labored breathing, and a compromised ability to forage or hunt. Burrowing species may face additional challenges as particles settle in underground habitats.

Aquatic Dwellers Under Threat: Aquatic wildlife, including fish and amphibians, confront respiratory challenges as PM2.5 particles settle on water surfaces. Gills of fish and amphibians may be adversely affected, compromising oxygen uptake and leading to physiological stress. Aquatic species sensitive to changes in water quality face increased vulnerability.

Behavioral Disruptions: Navigating the Animal Kingdom's Response

Altered Foraging Patterns: The introduction of PM2.5 into natural habitats can disrupt wildlife foraging behaviors. Species relying on olfactory cues to locate prey or identify suitable food sources may experience difficulties due to impaired air quality. Changes in foraging patterns can have cascading effects on predator-prey dynamics.

Migratory Challenges: Migratory species, often traversing vast distances, may encounter PM2.5 pollution along their migration routes. The impact on navigation, respiratory health, and energy expenditure during migration poses additional challenges for species dependent on successful journeys for their survival and reproduction.

Impact on Reproductive Strategies: Fine particulate matter can influence the reproductive strategies of wildlife. Changes in behavior, altered hormonal regulation, and compromised fertility may be observed. Nesting birds, in particular, may face challenges as PM2.5 settles on nests and affects incubation conditions.

Disruption of Communication: Wildlife relies on various forms of communication, including vocalizations, visual displays, and chemical signals. PM2.5 pollution can disrupt these communication channels, leading to misunderstandings among individuals. Species dependent on communication for mating rituals, territory defense, or group coordination may face challenges.

Cumulative Health Effects: Unraveling Long-Term Consequences

Chronic Health Impacts: The chronic exposure of wildlife to elevated levels of PM2.5 contributes to long-term health consequences. Respiratory diseases, compromised immune function, and reproductive issues may manifest over time, affecting individual fitness and the overall health of populations.

Population Dynamics: Changes in individual health can influence population dynamics. Reduced reproductive success, increased mortality rates, and altered age structures may be observed in wildlife populations exposed to persistent PM2.5 pollution. The long-term viability of species may be threatened, posing conservation challenges.

Interactions with Other Stressors: Wildlife often contends with multiple stressors, including habitat loss, climate change, and pollution. The interaction between PM2.5 pollution and other stressors can amplify the challenges faced by wildlife, creating synergistic effects that exacerbate the vulnerability of species.

Adaptation and Resilience: A Glimmer of Hope in the Wild

Natural Adaptations: Some wildlife species may exhibit natural adaptations to cope with environmental stressors, including PM2.5 pollution. Physiological changes, alterations in behavior, and genetic adaptations may confer a degree of resilience, allowing certain species to persist in polluted environments.

Behavioral Shifts: Wildlife can exhibit behavioral shifts in response to environmental challenges. Changes in habitat use, altered activity patterns, and shifts in daily routines may represent adaptive strategies aimed at minimizing exposure to PM2.5 and optimizing survival in human-altered landscapes.

Genetic Diversity and Evolution: Over time, the selective pressures exerted by PM2.5 pollution may influence genetic diversity within wildlife populations. Evolutionary processes may favor individuals with traits that enhance resilience to pollution, contributing to the genetic adaptation of wildlife over generations.

Species-Specific Vulnerabilities: A Diverse Canvas of Impact

Avian Vulnerabilities: Birds, with their diverse ecological roles and adaptations, face a range of vulnerabilities. Raptors, with their high-energy demands and dependence on keen eyesight, may be particularly affected. Ground-nesting birds and those relying on specific plant species for nesting materials may encounter challenges.

Mammalian Challenges: Terrestrial mammals exhibit varied vulnerabilities. Arboreal species, dependent on forest canopies, may face challenges due to settled particles on leaves and branches. Burrowing mammals, with habitats closer to ground level, may be directly exposed to airborne PM2.5.

Aquatic Susceptibilities: Aquatic species, residing in rivers, lakes, and oceans, experience unique susceptibilities. Fish with gill-based respiration may be directly impacted by waterborne PM2.5, while marine mammals surfacing for breath may inhale particles from the air. Amphibians, with permeable skin, may absorb pollutants directly.

Conservation Dilemmas: Balancing Preservation and Urbanization

Protected Areas Under Threat: Wildlife residing in protected areas, intended to serve as sanctuaries for biodiversity, may still face the encroachment of PM2.5 pollution. Human activities near reserves, industrial development, and transportation corridors can compromise the integrity of protected habitats.

Urban Wildlife Challenges: Species adapted to urban environments, often characterized by higher levels of PM2.5 pollution, face a different set of challenges. Urban wildlife, including birds, rodents, and insects, may display unique adaptations but can also experience health impacts and altered behavior due to pollution exposure.

Conservation Strategies for Urban Wildlife: Implementing conservation strategies for urban wildlife involves a nuanced approach. Green spaces, habitat restoration, and pollution mitigation measures in urban areas contribute to creating environments where wildlife can coexist with human activities.

Global Perspectives: Wildlife in a Changing World

Transboundary Impact: PM2.5 pollution, with its ability to travel across borders, poses a transboundary challenge for wildlife. Migratory species, spanning continents and oceans, may encounter pollution from distant sources. Addressing the global impact on wildlife requires international cooperation and shared conservation efforts.

Cross-Species Implications: The impact of PM2.5 on wildlife extends beyond individual species. Interconnected ecosystems involve intricate relationships between species, and disruptions caused by pollution can have cascading effects. Conserving biodiversity requires a holistic understanding of these interactions.

Climate Change and Wildlife Vulnerability: The interactions between PM2.5 pollution and climate change further complicate the challenges faced by wildlife. Changes in temperature, precipitation patterns, and habitat distribution interact with pollution-induced stressors, amplifying the vulnerability of species to environmental changes.

Conclusion: Navigating Wildlife Challenges

As we navigate the complex challenges faced by wildlife in the wake of PM2.5 pollution, a profound understanding of the diverse vulnerabilities and adaptive strategies emerges. The journey toward mitigating the impact on wildlife involves not only unraveling the intricacies of these challenges but also fostering a collective commitment to creating environments where every species, from the tiniest insects to the largest predators, can thrive and endure.

In the chapters that follow, we will delve into specific case studies, success stories, and ongoing challenges related to the effects of PM2.5 on wildlife, aiming to unravel the complexities of managing air pollution on a global scale. The journey towards cleaner air involves not only acknowledging the ecological consequences but also fostering a collective commitment to creating a world where wildlife coexists harmoniously with the pervasive influence of fine particulate matter.

Soil and Water Contamination

As PM2.5 pollution infiltrates the air we breathe, its insidious effects extend beyond the atmosphere, permeating the very soil beneath our feet and the water bodies that sustain life. This chapter delves into the intricate pathways through which fine particulate matter contaminates soil and water, unraveling the consequences for ecosystems, agriculture, and human well-being.

The Unseen Intruder: PM2.5 in Earth's Elemental Reservoirs

Soil and water, essential components of Earth's ecosystems, act as repositories of life-sustaining elements. The introduction of PM2.5 pollution into these vital resources disrupts the delicate balance of nutrients, alters the chemistry of soils and water bodies, and poses a range of challenges that echo through terrestrial and aquatic ecosystems.

Soil Contamination: Disrupting the Ground Beneath

Deposition Mechanisms: PM2.5 particles settle on the Earth's surface through various deposition mechanisms, including dry deposition and wet deposition. Dry deposition involves the direct settling of particles from the air onto soil surfaces, while wet deposition involves the deposition of particles carried by rain or other forms of precipitation.

Chemical Composition of PM2.5: The chemical composition of PM2.5 plays a crucial role in soil contamination. Fine particulate matter may carry heavy metals, organic compounds, and other pollutants. Once deposited on soil, these components can influence soil chemistry, nutrient availability, and the health of soil-dwelling organisms.

Effects on Soil Structure: The accumulation of PM2.5 particles in soil can alter its physical structure. Fine particulate matter may contribute to soil compaction, reducing porosity and water infiltration. Changes in soil structure can impact root growth, nutrient uptake, and the overall fertility of agricultural and natural ecosystems.

Nutrient Imbalance: PM2.5 pollution can introduce imbalances in soil nutrient availability. The deposition of pollutants may lead to elevated levels of certain elements, such as heavy metals, while depleting essential nutrients. This imbalance affects plant growth, disrupts nutrient cycling, and poses challenges for agriculture and ecosystem health.

Agricultural Impacts: Crop Health and Food Security Concerns

Crop Contamination: PM2.5 pollution poses a risk to agricultural crops through soil contamination. Fine particulate matter can deposit on plant surfaces, and the subsequent absorption of pollutants can affect crop quality. The accumulation of heavy metals in edible parts of plants raises concerns for food safety and human health.

Reduced Crop Yields: Soil contamination with PM2.5 may contribute to reduced crop yields. Changes in soil fertility, nutrient imbalances, and the direct impact of pollutants on plant physiology can result in lower agricultural productivity. This poses challenges for global food security, especially in regions with high levels of air pollution.

Impacts on Soil Microbes: Soil-dwelling microbes play a crucial role in nutrient cycling, organic matter decomposition, and the overall health of soils. PM2.5 pollution can affect the composition and activity of soil microbial communities, disrupting essential ecosystem processes and compromising soil resilience.

Water Runoff and Contamination: Fine particulate matter deposited on soil surfaces can be transported by water runoff, contributing to water contamination. The runoff may carry pollutants into rivers, lakes, and other water bodies, affecting aquatic ecosystems and posing risks for human consumption of contaminated water.

Water Contamination: The Silent Infiltration

Aquatic Deposition: PM2.5 pollution reaches water bodies through atmospheric deposition. Rainwater carries settled particles into rivers, lakes, and oceans, introducing pollutants into aquatic ecosystems. The proximity of water bodies to pollution sources, such as industrial areas and urban centers, amplifies the risk of water contamination.

Sediment Accumulation: Fine particulate matter settles in aquatic sediments, accumulating over time. The deposition of PM2.5 in sediments raises concerns for the long-term contamination of aquatic ecosystems. Sediments act as reservoirs for pollutants, releasing them back into the water column and affecting the health of aquatic organisms.

Impact on Aquatic Organisms: Water contamination with PM2.5 poses risks for aquatic organisms. Fish, invertebrates, and other aquatic species may be exposed to pollutants through water ingestion, gill respiration, and the consumption of contaminated prey. The physiological health, reproductive success, and survival of aquatic organisms may be compromised.

Altered Water Chemistry: The introduction of PM2.5 pollutants into water bodies can alter water chemistry. Changes in pH, nutrient levels, and the concentration of heavy metals can impact the composition of aquatic communities. Altered water chemistry poses challenges for the maintenance of healthy aquatic ecosystems.

Ecosystem Resilience: Navigating the Contaminated Landscape

Bioaccumulation and Biomagnification: PM2.5 pollutants can undergo bioaccumulation and biomagnification in aquatic ecosystems. This process involves the accumulation of pollutants in the tissues of aquatic organisms, with higher trophic levels experiencing elevated concentrations. Predatory species, including fish and birds, may face increased risks.

Impact on Aquatic Plants: Aquatic plants play a vital role in maintaining water quality by contributing to oxygen production and nutrient cycling. PM2.5 pollution can affect the health of aquatic plants through direct exposure to settled particles and changes in water chemistry. Altered plant communities may impact the overall structure of aquatic ecosystems.

Wetland Ecosystems Under Threat: Wetlands, acting as crucial ecological filters, may face threats from PM2.5 pollution. The deposition of pollutants in wetland areas can disrupt the functions of these ecosystems, affecting water purification, habitat provision, and the overall resilience of wetland communities.

Groundwater Contamination: PM2.5 pollutants can percolate through soil and reach groundwater, contributing to groundwater contamination. The infiltration of pollutants into aquifers raises concerns for the quality of drinking water supplies and poses challenges for mitigating contamination in subsurface environments.

Human Health Concerns: Tracing the Pathways

Contaminated Food Supply: Soil contamination with PM2.5 poses risks for human health through the consumption of contaminated crops. The bioaccumulation of pollutants in edible plant parts, such as fruits and vegetables, raises concerns for exposure to heavy metals and other contaminants through the food supply.

Drinking Water Hazards: Water contamination with PM2.5 pollutants poses hazards for human health through the consumption of contaminated drinking water. The infiltration of pollutants into groundwater and surface water sources creates challenges for ensuring safe drinking water supplies, especially in regions with high pollution levels.

Respiratory and Dermatological Effects: Dust resuspension from contaminated soil surfaces can contribute to elevated PM2.5 levels in the air. This poses risks for respiratory and dermatological effects as individuals may inhale or come into contact with contaminated dust particles. Skin irritation, respiratory distress, and other health issues may result.

Urbanization and Exposure Risks: Urban areas, characterized by higher levels of PM2.5 pollution, may face increased risks of soil and water contamination. The proximity of pollution sources, industrial activities, and traffic emissions amplifies the exposure risks for urban populations, highlighting the importance of pollution mitigation in densely populated areas.

Mitigation Strategies: Balancing Earth's Elemental Equation

Soil Remediation Techniques: Mitigating soil contamination involves the application of remediation techniques. These may include phytoremediation, where plants are used to absorb and accumulate pollutants, and soil amendments to enhance nutrient availability and soil structure. Sustainable agricultural practices contribute to minimizing soil contamination risks.

Water Treatment Measures: Managing water contamination with PM2.5 pollutants requires effective water treatment measures. Filtration, sedimentation, and chemical treatment processes can be employed to remove fine particulate matter from water sources. Protecting natural buffer zones, such as wetlands, contributes to reducing contamination risks.

Policy Interventions: Addressing soil and water contamination from PM2.5 pollution necessitates policy interventions at local, national, and international levels. Implementing and enforcing regulations on industrial emissions, promoting sustainable land use practices, and investing in pollution control technologies contribute to minimizing contamination risks.

Community Engagement and Education: Involving communities in pollution monitoring, promoting awareness of contamination risks, and encouraging sustainable practices contribute to mitigating the impacts of PM2.5 pollution on soil and water. Education campaigns on proper waste disposal, responsible chemical use, and sustainable agriculture empower individuals to contribute to pollution prevention.

Global Collaboration: Safeguarding Earth's Elemental Reservoirs

Transboundary Pollution Management: PM2.5 pollution, with its ability to travel across regions and borders, requires global collaboration. Transboundary pollution management involves international agreements, shared research initiatives, and coordinated efforts to address the sources and consequences of fine particulate matter on a planetary scale.

Research and Monitoring: Advancing scientific research and monitoring programs contribute to a deeper understanding of the pathways and impacts of PM2.5 pollution on soil and water. Robust monitoring systems facilitate the tracking of pollution sources, assessing contamination levels, and guiding mitigation efforts.

Climate Change Adaptation: The interactions between PM2.5 pollution, soil and water contamination, and climate change underscore the need for integrated approaches to environmental management. Adaptation strategies that consider the interconnected nature of these challenges contribute to building resilient ecosystems and safeguarding Earth's elemental reservoirs.

Conclusion: Balancing the Elemental Equation

As we navigate the complexities of soil and water contamination from PM2.5 pollution, a profound realization emerges—that the health of Earth's elemental reservoirs is intricately linked to the well-being of ecosystems, agriculture, and human societies. The journey toward cleaner air involves not only mitigating the atmospheric presence of fine particulate matter but also fostering a collective commitment to safeguarding the essential elements that sustain life on our planet.

In the chapters that follow, we will delve into specific case studies, success stories, and ongoing challenges related to soil and water contamination, aiming to unravel the complexities of managing PM2.5 pollution on a global scale. The journey towards cleaner air involves not only acknowledging the environmental consequences but also fostering a collective commitment to creating a world where soil and water thrive, unperturbed by the silent creep of fine particulate matter.

Interconnectedness with Climate Change

In the intricate web of Earth's environmental dynamics, the influence of PM2.5 pollution extends beyond the immediate consequences on air quality, soil, and water. This chapter explores the interconnectedness between fine particulate matter and climate change, unraveling the symbiotic dance that shapes the destiny of our planet's atmospheric and ecological equilibrium.

Atmospheric Dynamics: PM2.5 as Climate Actors

The presence of PM2.5 particles in the atmosphere goes beyond their role as mere pollutants; these fine particles actively participate in the intricate dance of climate dynamics, influencing temperature patterns, precipitation regimes, and atmospheric stability.

Radiative Forcing: The Climate Impact of PM2.5

Absorption and Scattering: PM2.5 particles have distinct properties that influence their interaction with solar radiation. While some particles absorb sunlight, contributing to local warming, others scatter sunlight back into space. This dual role of absorption and scattering collectively influences radiative forcing, contributing to regional and global climate effects.

Albedo Modification: The presence of PM2.5 particles in the atmosphere can alter surface albedo—the reflectivity of Earth's surface. Dark particles, such as those containing black carbon, absorb more sunlight, leading to localized warming. Changes in albedo contribute to regional climate variations and impact ecosystems, particularly those adapted to specific temperature ranges.

Regional Climate Effects: PM2.5-induced radiative forcing can result in regional climate effects. The warming or cooling of specific regions influences atmospheric circulation patterns, impacting weather systems, and contributing to phenomena such as heatwaves, droughts, or altered precipitation patterns. These effects add an additional layer of complexity to the interconnected relationship between PM2.5 and climate dynamics.

Feedback Loops: Amplifying Environmental Changes

Ice-Albedo Feedback: In polar regions, where ice and snow cover vast expanses, PM2.5 pollution can accelerate ice melt through the ice-albedo feedback loop. Dark particles settling on ice surfaces absorb sunlight, leading to increased melting. As ice melts, the surface becomes darker, further enhancing the absorption of sunlight—a self-reinforcing loop with implications for sea-level rise.

Land Use Changes: The impact of PM2.5 pollution on ecosystems and agriculture can contribute to land use changes. Deforestation, altered vegetation patterns, and shifts in land cover influence the Earth's energy balance and contribute to feedback loops that amplify climate change. These changes may result in altered precipitation patterns and disruptions to regional climates.

Ocean-Atmosphere Interactions: PM2.5 particles can influence ocean-atmosphere interactions, particularly in regions with high pollution levels. Aerosols can serve as cloud condensation nuclei, affecting cloud formation and properties. Changes in cloud cover, precipitation, and atmospheric circulation patterns contribute to complex feedback loops that influence regional and global climates.

Global Circulation Changes: The interconnectedness between PM2.5 pollution and climate change extends to global circulation patterns. The alteration of temperature gradients, atmospheric stability, and pressure systems influences the behavior of jet streams and other major wind patterns. These changes have cascading effects on weather systems, storm tracks, and climate variability.

Impacts on Carbon Cycles: PM2.5 pollution can influence carbon cycles in terrestrial and aquatic ecosystems. Changes in plant productivity, soil respiration, and carbon sequestration may result from the direct and indirect impacts of fine particulate matter. Alterations in carbon cycles contribute to climate feedback loops, influencing greenhouse gas concentrations in the atmosphere.

Sea Level Rise and Glacial Retreat: The influence of PM2.5 pollution on climate dynamics contributes to sea level rise and glacial retreat. Warming temperatures, altered precipitation patterns, and the acceleration of ice melt in polar and glacial regions collectively contribute to changes in global sea levels, impacting coastal ecosystems and human communities.

Climate Change and Pollution Sources: A Two-Way Street

The relationship between climate change and PM2.5 pollution is not unidirectional; it is a dynamic interaction where climate change influences pollution sources, and pollution, in turn, contributes to climate variability. This intricate interplay highlights the importance of considering the broader environmental context when addressing the consequences of fine particulate matter on our planet.

Climate-Induced Changes in Pollution Sources

Wildfires and Biomass Burning: Climate change can influence the frequency and intensity of wildfires, contributing to increased emissions of PM2.5 particles from biomass burning. Extended fire seasons, altered vegetation patterns, and drier conditions create favorable conditions for wildfires, releasing large amounts of fine particulate matter into the atmosphere.

Changing Meteorological Patterns: Climate change affects meteorological patterns, including temperature, precipitation, and wind regimes. These changes influence the dispersion, transformation, and deposition of pollutants in the atmosphere. Altered meteorological patterns may contribute to the spatial and temporal distribution of PM2.5 pollution, impacting air quality on regional and global scales.

Exacerbation of Natural Sources: Climate change can exacerbate natural sources of PM2.5 pollution. Dust storms, volcanic eruptions, and biogenic emissions may become more frequent or intense under changing climate conditions. The increased contribution of natural sources adds complexity to the overall burden of fine particulate matter in the atmosphere.

Anthropogenic Contributions to Climate Change

Carbon Emissions and Black Carbon: The combustion of fossil fuels, a major contributor to climate change, releases not only greenhouse gases but also black carbon—a component of PM2.5 pollution. Black carbon, with its strong light-absorbing properties, contributes to regional warming and influences climate dynamics, particularly in areas with high concentrations of pollution.

Methane and Short-Lived Climate Pollutants: Anthropogenic sources of methane and other short-lived climate pollutants contribute to climate change and influence the atmospheric composition. The interaction between these pollutants and PM2.5 particles can have complex effects on radiative forcing, atmospheric chemistry, and regional climates, highlighting the interconnected nature of air quality and climate dynamics.

Feedbacks from Industrial Activities: Industrial processes, another major source of both air pollution and greenhouse gas emissions, contribute to the complex interplay between PM2.5 pollution and climate change. The emissions of particulate matter, gases, and aerosols from industrial activities can influence cloud formation, precipitation patterns, and regional climates, creating feedback loops that amplify environmental changes.

Climate Change Mitigation and Air Quality Co-Benefits

Recognizing the interconnectedness of climate change and PM2.5 pollution opens avenues for integrated strategies that address both challenges simultaneously. Climate change mitigation measures can lead to air quality co-benefits, fostering a holistic approach to environmental management.

Transition to Renewable Energy: Shifting from fossil fuel-based energy sources to renewable alternatives contributes to reducing greenhouse gas emissions and mitigating climate change. Simultaneously, this transition reduces the emissions of particulate matter and other air pollutants, improving air quality and public health.

Sustainable Transportation: Promoting sustainable transportation modes, such as electric vehicles, cycling, and public transit, not only reduces carbon emissions but also curtails air pollution from vehicular sources. Integrated urban planning that prioritizes walkable and bike-friendly environments further contributes to both climate and air quality goals.

Afforestation and Green Spaces: Afforestation initiatives, aimed at increasing forest cover and restoring green spaces, contribute to carbon sequestration and climate change mitigation. Additionally, trees and greenery act as natural filters, reducing the concentration of PM2.5 particles in the air and improving local air quality.

Energy Efficiency and Pollution Control Technologies: Enhancing energy efficiency in industrial processes and implementing pollution control technologies not only reduces greenhouse gas emissions but also minimizes the release of particulate matter and other pollutants. These measures offer dual benefits by addressing both climate change and air quality concerns.

Integrated Policy Approaches: Implementing integrated policy approaches that consider both climate change and air quality objectives is essential. Coordinated efforts at local, national, and international levels can leverage synergies between climate change mitigation strategies and air quality improvement measures, fostering a comprehensive and sustainable approach to environmental management.

Global Perspectives: Addressing Interconnected Challenges

The interconnectedness between PM2.5 pollution and climate change transcends geographical boundaries, requiring collaborative efforts on a global scale. Addressing the challenges posed by these intertwined environmental issues necessitates international cooperation, shared research endeavors, and coordinated actions to safeguard the health of our planet.

International Agreements: Existing international agreements, such as the Paris Agreement, acknowledge the interlinkages between air quality, climate change, and sustainable development. Strengthening and expanding such agreements contribute to a unified global approach to addressing the complex challenges posed by fine particulate matter and climate variability.

Research Collaborations: Advancing scientific research and collaborations on the interactions between PM2.5 pollution and climate change is essential. Research initiatives that span disciplines, engage diverse stakeholders, and leverage emerging technologies contribute to a deeper understanding of the complex dynamics at play.

Climate and Air Quality Monitoring: Robust monitoring systems for both climate parameters and air quality provide critical data for informed decision-making. Integrated monitoring networks contribute to tracking the impacts of PM2.5 pollution on climate and vice versa, guiding policy interventions, and assessing the effectiveness of mitigation measures.

Community Engagement and Awareness: Involving communities in the dialogue on interconnected environmental challenges fosters a sense of shared responsibility. Raising awareness of the links between PM2.5 pollution and climate change empowers individuals to contribute to local and global efforts, promoting sustainable practices and advocating for pollution reduction measures.

Education and Capacity Building: Education programs and capacity-building initiatives play a pivotal role in addressing interconnected environmental challenges. Equipping individuals, communities, and policymakers with the knowledge and tools to understand and navigate the complexities of PM2.5 pollution and climate change contributes to building resilience and fostering adaptive strategies.

Conclusion: Navigating the Interconnected Horizon

As we navigate the interconnected horizon of PM2.5 pollution and climate change, a profound realization emerges—that the health of our planet's atmosphere, ecosystems, and human societies is woven into a tapestry of interdependence. The journey toward cleaner air involves not only mitigating the immediate impacts of fine particulate matter but also fostering a collective commitment to addressing the broader environmental challenges that shape the destiny of our shared home.

In the chapters that follow, we will delve into specific case studies, success stories, and ongoing challenges related to the interconnectedness between PM2.5 pollution and climate change. The journey towards cleaner air involves not only acknowledging the complex dynamics at play but also fostering a collective commitment to creating a world where the dance between fine particulate matter and climate variability is harmonious and sustainable.

Chapter 5: Government Policies and Regulations

Overview of Existing Policies

In the face of the escalating challenge posed by PM2.5 pollution, governments worldwide have implemented a spectrum of policies and regulations aimed at curbing emissions, improving air quality, and safeguarding public health. This section provides an in-depth overview of the existing policies, exploring the diverse approaches governments have taken to address the multifaceted dimensions of fine particulate matter pollution.

National Air Quality Standards: Establishing Baselines for Air Quality

Defining Acceptable Limits: Many countries have established National Ambient Air Quality Standards (NAAQS) that set permissible limits for various air pollutants, including PM2.5. These standards serve as benchmarks to assess the concentration of fine particulate matter in the air and guide regulatory efforts to maintain or achieve acceptable air quality levels.

Variable Standards Across Countries: The specific standards vary significantly from country to country, reflecting differences in environmental conditions, industrialization levels, and public health priorities. Some nations adopt stringent standards to protect vulnerable populations, while others may face challenges in implementation due to economic considerations or resource constraints.

Emission Standards for Industries: Targeting Pollution Sources

Sector-Specific Regulations: Governments often implement emission standards that target specific industries and sources of pollution. These regulations establish limits on the amount of PM2.5 and other pollutants that industries are permitted to release into the air. Sectors such as power plants, manufacturing facilities, and transportation are commonly subject to such standards.

Technological Requirements: Emission standards may prescribe the use of specific technologies, such as particulate matter filters, scrubbers, or cleaner fuel technologies, to reduce the release of fine particulate matter. The adoption of cleaner technologies not only mitigates air pollution but also contributes to improving overall industrial sustainability.

Vehicle Emission Standards: Tackling Mobile Sources

Stringent Vehicle Standards: Transportation, a significant contributor to PM2.5 pollution, is often targeted through vehicle emission standards. Governments establish limits on the amount of particulate matter that vehicles, including cars, trucks, and buses, are allowed to emit. These standards encourage the adoption of cleaner engines and exhaust control technologies.

Transition to Electric and Alternative Fuels: Some countries emphasize the transition to electric vehicles and alternative fuels as part of their vehicle emission control strategies. Incentives for electric vehicles, the development of charging infrastructure, and the promotion of public transportation contribute to reducing emissions from the transportation sector.

Regional and Local Measures: Tailoring Solutions to Specific Contexts

Geographically Tailored Policies: In regions with distinct air quality challenges, governments may implement geographically tailored policies. These could include specific regulations for urban areas with high pollution levels, measures to address pollution hotspots, or targeted interventions in regions with unique sources of fine particulate matter.

City-Level Initiatives: Many cities worldwide have adopted localized measures to combat PM2.5 pollution. These initiatives may include restrictions on vehicle use, the promotion of green spaces, and the implementation of urban planning strategies to reduce pollution concentrations in densely populated areas.

Cap-and-Trade Systems: Economic Instruments for Pollution Reduction

Market-Based Approaches: Some countries have embraced market-based mechanisms, such as cap-and-trade systems, to control emissions. These systems set an overall cap on the total amount of pollutants, including PM2.5, that can be released by covered entities. Companies are then allocated or purchase permits, creating economic incentives for emission reductions.

Flexibility and Innovation: Cap-and-trade systems offer flexibility for businesses to find cost-effective ways to reduce emissions. This market-oriented approach encourages innovation in pollution control technologies and provides a framework for achieving emissions reductions while supporting economic growth.

International Agreements: Collaborative Efforts on a Global Scale

Global Cooperation: Recognizing the transboundary nature of air pollution, countries engage in international agreements to address PM2.5 pollution collectively. Agreements such as the Convention on Long-Range Transboundary Air Pollution (CLRTAP) and the Paris Agreement underscore the importance of global collaboration to mitigate the impacts of fine particulate matter on air quality and climate.

Shared Research and Data Exchange: International agreements often include provisions for shared research initiatives, data exchange, and collaborative efforts to understand the sources, transport, and impacts of PM2.5 pollution. This collective knowledge contributes to informed policy decisions and enhances the effectiveness of mitigation strategies on a global scale.

Public Awareness and Education: Empowering Communities

Community Engagement: Governments recognize the importance of engaging communities in the fight against PM2.5 pollution. Public awareness campaigns, educational programs, and community initiatives empower individuals to understand the sources and health impacts of fine particulate matter, encouraging collective action for cleaner air.

Citizen Science: Some countries leverage citizen science initiatives, where members of the public actively contribute to air quality monitoring efforts. This bottom-up approach not only expands the coverage of monitoring networks but also fosters a sense of shared responsibility, making communities active participants in the quest for cleaner air.

Challenges and Opportunities: Navigating the Policy Landscape

Implementation Challenges: While many countries have instituted policies to address PM2.5 pollution, the effective implementation of these measures often faces challenges. These challenges may include resource constraints, regulatory enforcement issues, and the need for coordinated efforts across different sectors and levels of government.

Integration with Climate Policies: The interconnected nature of PM2.5 pollution and climate change highlights the importance of integrating air quality policies with broader climate mitigation and adaptation strategies. Governments face opportunities to leverage synergies between environmental goals and develop holistic approaches to address interconnected challenges.

Technological Advancements: Advancements in technology offer opportunities for more effective and targeted policies. Continuous improvements in air quality monitoring technologies, pollution control devices, and data analytics provide governments with the tools to refine and adapt their policies for better outcomes.

Conclusion: Charting the Course Forward

As we navigate the policy landscape for PM2.5 pollution, a complex tapestry of regulations, incentives, and collaborative efforts emerges. Governments worldwide are grappling with the challenge of balancing economic development with the imperative to safeguard air quality and public health. The journey towards cleaner air involves not only the creation of effective policies but also their vigilant implementation, continuous evaluation, and adaptation to meet evolving environmental challenges.

In the chapters that follow, we will delve into specific case studies, success stories, and ongoing challenges related to government policies and regulations for PM2.5 pollution. The journey towards cleaner air involves not only navigating the intricacies of existing policies but also fostering a collective commitment to shaping a future where the air we breathe is a testament to the success of thoughtful and impactful regulations.

International Collaboration Efforts

In the global pursuit of cleaner air and the mitigation of PM2.5 pollution, the interconnected nature of air quality challenges necessitates collaborative efforts across borders. International cooperation brings together governments, organizations, and experts to share knowledge, resources, and strategies. This section explores the diverse avenues of international collaboration, highlighting the significance of unified action in addressing the transboundary impacts of fine particulate matter.

Global Understanding: Shared Research Initiatives

Transboundary Air Pollution Research: Recognizing the need for a comprehensive understanding of PM2.5 pollution, international collaborative efforts often involve shared research initiatives. Studies on the transboundary transport of fine particulate matter, its sources, and its impacts on air quality and climate contribute to a global knowledge base.

Monitoring Networks: Collaborative monitoring networks facilitate the collection of data on PM2.5 concentrations, emission sources, and atmospheric dynamics across different regions. These networks, often established through international agreements, provide valuable insights into the spatial and temporal variations of fine particulate matter, guiding policy interventions.

Data Exchange and Standardization: The exchange of air quality data among countries allows for a more comprehensive analysis of pollution patterns. Standardizing measurement methods and data reporting practices enhances the comparability of information, supporting accurate assessments of PM2.5 levels and facilitating the development of effective mitigation strategies.

International Agreements: Frameworks for Collective Action

Convention on Long-Range Transboundary Air Pollution (CLRTAP): The CLRTAP, under the auspices of the United Nations Economic Commission for Europe (UNECE), stands as a pioneering international agreement addressing transboundary air pollution, including PM2.5. Adopted in 1979, the convention fosters cooperation among countries to reduce air pollution and its adverse effects.

Protocols and Amendments: The CLRTAP includes protocols that focus on specific pollutants, such as sulfur dioxide (SO_2), nitrogen oxides (NO_x), and particulate matter. Protocols related to PM2.5 aim to limit emissions and establish reduction targets. Amendments to existing protocols reflect evolving scientific knowledge and emerging challenges, providing a flexible framework for collective action.

Implementation Mechanisms: The convention and its protocols incorporate mechanisms for the implementation of agreed-upon measures. These mechanisms may involve periodic reporting, emission inventories, and compliance assessment. By fostering transparency and accountability, the CLRTAP enhances the effectiveness of international efforts to address PM2.5 pollution.

Paris Agreement: A Holistic Approach to Environmental Challenges

Climate Change and Air Quality Linkages: The Paris Agreement, adopted in 2015, recognizes the interconnectedness between climate change and air quality. While primarily focused on mitigating climate change, the agreement acknowledges the co-benefits of climate action for air quality improvement, aligning with efforts to address the impacts of PM2.5 pollution.

Nationally Determined Contributions (NDCs): Countries participating in the Paris Agreement submit NDCs outlining their climate action plans. Some NDCs include commitments related to reducing air pollutants, including PM2.5. By integrating air quality considerations into climate strategies, nations contribute to both environmental goals.

Synergies with Sustainable Development Goals (SDGs): The Paris Agreement aligns with the United Nations Sustainable Development Goals (SDGs), creating synergies between climate action, air quality improvement, and broader socioeconomic objectives. This integrated approach reflects the understanding that addressing PM2.5 pollution requires multifaceted and collaborative solutions.

Bilateral and Regional Partnerships: Tailoring Solutions to Regions

Bilateral Agreements: Countries often engage in bilateral agreements to address shared air quality challenges. These agreements may involve joint research projects, technology transfer, and collaborative initiatives to reduce cross-border pollution. Bilateral efforts allow nations to tailor solutions to their specific circumstances and priorities.

Regional Cooperation: Asia-Pacific Partnership on Clean Development and Climate (APP): Regional partnerships, such as the APP, bring together countries facing common air quality challenges. The APP focuses on clean development, technology transfer, and capacity-building to address air pollution and climate change in the Asia-Pacific region. Regional collaboration fosters the exchange of best practices and shared solutions.

European Union (EU) Initiatives: Within the European Union, efforts to combat air pollution extend beyond national borders. The EU's Ambient Air Quality Directive sets standards for PM2.5 concentrations, and collaborative initiatives, such as the European Green Deal, emphasize cross-border cooperation to improve air quality and reduce emissions.

Emergency Response and Early Warning Systems: Timely Alerts Across Borders

Transboundary Pollution Episodes: In cases of severe air pollution episodes, especially those involving transboundary transport of pollutants, early warning systems are crucial. Collaborative efforts to establish effective communication channels and alert mechanisms ensure timely responses to emerging air quality challenges, protecting public health across borders.

Information Sharing and Coordination: International collaboration enables the sharing of information on pollution sources, meteorological conditions, and potential transboundary impacts. Coordinated responses, including public advisories, temporary regulatory measures, and cross-border cooperation on emergency interventions, help mitigate the consequences of severe pollution episodes.

Capacity Building and Technical Assistance: Empowering Nations

Knowledge Transfer: International collaboration includes initiatives for knowledge transfer and capacity building. Experienced countries assist others in developing and implementing effective air quality management strategies. This transfer of knowledge encompasses technological expertise, policy development, and the establishment of monitoring and regulatory frameworks.

Technical Assistance Programs: Organizations and initiatives, such as the World Bank's Clean Air Fund, provide technical assistance and financial support to countries striving to improve air quality. These programs assist in the development of emission inventories, air quality monitoring networks, and the implementation of effective regulatory measures.

Challenges and Opportunities: Navigating the Complex Terrain

Harmonizing Diverse Approaches: The diversity of political, economic, and environmental contexts among countries poses challenges to harmonizing approaches to address PM2.5 pollution. Bridging gaps in policies, standards, and implementation strategies requires ongoing dialogue and a commitment to shared goals.

Funding and Resource Disparities: Disparities in funding and technical resources among nations can hinder effective collaboration. Initiatives that address resource gaps, facilitate technology transfer, and prioritize the needs of developing countries contribute to building a more equitable and impactful collaborative framework.

Political Will and Commitment: The success of international collaboration efforts hinges on the political will and commitment of participating countries. Sustained efforts to foster a shared understanding of the urgency of addressing PM2.5 pollution, along with the recognition of its interconnected impacts, contribute to the resilience and effectiveness of collaborative initiatives.

Conclusion: Forging a Global Alliance Against PM2.5 Pollution

As we delve into the complexities of international collaboration efforts against PM2.5 pollution, a clear narrative emerges—one of shared responsibility, mutual understanding, and the recognition that the air we breathe knows no borders. The journey towards cleaner air involves not only the implementation of effective policies at the national level but also a commitment to collective action on the global stage.

In the chapters that follow, we will explore specific case studies, success stories, and ongoing challenges related to international collaboration efforts. The journey towards cleaner air involves not only navigating the complex terrain of global partnerships but also fostering a collective commitment to creating a world where the fight against PM2.5 pollution transcends borders and unites nations in a common pursuit of air quality excellence.

Challenges in Implementation

As nations endeavor to combat PM2.5 pollution through government policies and regulations, the path to implementation is fraught with challenges. From resource constraints to regulatory enforcement issues, understanding and addressing these challenges are pivotal for the success of air quality initiatives. This section explores the multifaceted hurdles encountered in the implementation of policies aimed at mitigating the impacts of fine particulate matter.

Resource Constraints: Balancing Economic Development and Environmental Goals

Financial Limitations: One of the primary challenges in implementing robust air quality policies is the financial burden associated with adopting and enforcing regulations. Many countries, particularly those in the developing world, face resource constraints that limit their capacity to invest in advanced pollution control technologies, comprehensive monitoring networks, and the enforcement infrastructure needed to ensure compliance.

Technological Investments: The transition to cleaner technologies often requires substantial investments in research, development, and implementation. Industries may face financial barriers to upgrading their equipment or adopting cleaner processes. Governments need to strike a delicate balance between promoting economic development and safeguarding environmental quality, especially in regions where industries are significant contributors to the economy.

Enforcement and Regulatory Compliance: Bridging the Gap

Regulatory Ambiguities: Ambiguities in regulatory frameworks can hinder effective implementation. Vague or complex regulations may create challenges for industries in understanding compliance requirements. Clear and concise regulations, coupled with effective communication, are crucial for ensuring that businesses can align their practices with established air quality standards.

Regulatory Enforcement Gaps: Even with well-defined regulations, enforcement gaps pose a significant challenge. Inadequate monitoring, limited inspection capabilities, and a lack of resources for regulatory agencies can compromise the enforcement of air quality standards. Strengthening enforcement mechanisms through increased staffing, training, and the use of advanced monitoring technologies is essential to ensure compliance.

Data Collection and Monitoring: The Foundation of Effective Policies

Monitoring Infrastructure: Accurate and reliable data form the backbone of successful air quality policies. However, establishing and maintaining a robust monitoring infrastructure can be challenging, particularly in regions with limited resources. Investments in monitoring stations, air quality modeling, and data analysis capabilities are essential for obtaining a comprehensive understanding of PM2.5 concentrations.

Data Accessibility and Transparency: Accessibility to air quality data is critical for public awareness and stakeholder engagement. Challenges arise when data is not readily available, not easily understandable, or not transparent. Improving data accessibility through online platforms, real-time monitoring, and public reporting mechanisms enhances the effectiveness of air quality management.

Intersectoral Coordination: Breaking Silos for Holistic Solutions

Cross-Sectoral Collaboration: Addressing PM2.5 pollution requires collaboration across various sectors, including industry, transportation, urban planning, and health. Challenges arise when there is a lack of coordination between these sectors. Siloed approaches hinder the development and implementation of integrated solutions that consider the diverse sources of fine particulate matter.

Urban Planning and Transport Integration: In urban areas, the integration of air quality considerations into urban planning and transportation strategies is vital. Challenges emerge when urban development priorities do not align with air quality objectives. Implementing cohesive policies that prioritize sustainable urban design, public transportation, and green spaces requires coordination between city planners and environmental authorities.

Public Engagement and Awareness: Empowering Communities

Limited Public Awareness: Engaging the public in air quality management is challenging when there is limited awareness of the sources, health impacts, and potential mitigation measures related to PM2.5 pollution. Governments face the task of raising awareness through educational programs, outreach campaigns, and community involvement initiatives to ensure that individuals can make informed choices and advocate for cleaner air.

Community Involvement Gaps: Despite efforts to engage communities, gaps in community involvement may arise due to factors such as language barriers, socioeconomic disparities, or a lack of avenues for public participation. Bridging these gaps requires targeted outreach strategies, culturally sensitive communication, and the creation of platforms for meaningful community engagement in decision-making processes.

Political Will and Policy Consistency: Sustaining Commitment Over Time

Changing Political Priorities: Political will plays a crucial role in the success of air quality policies. Challenges emerge when political priorities shift, leading to a reduced emphasis on environmental concerns. Long-term commitment to air quality goals requires consistent support from policymakers and a recognition of the enduring impacts of PM2.5 pollution on public health and the environment.

Policy Consistency: Frequent changes in environmental policies and regulations can create uncertainty for industries and hinder long-term planning. Policy inconsistencies may result from shifts in government leadership or changing public sentiment. A stable regulatory environment that provides clear expectations and incentives for compliance is essential for fostering industry cooperation.

International Cooperation Challenges: Bridging Global Divides

Differing National Agendas: International collaboration faces challenges when countries prioritize their individual national agendas over collective efforts to combat PM2.5 pollution. Disparities in economic development, political priorities, and environmental regulations among nations may hinder the establishment of a unified global front against transboundary air pollution.

Equitable Participation: Ensuring equitable participation in international agreements and collaborations is essential. Developing countries, often facing resource constraints and pressing economic priorities, may find it challenging to actively engage in global initiatives. Bridging the gap requires a commitment to inclusive decision-making and mechanisms that support the participation of all nations.

Conclusion: Charting a Course Beyond Challenges

As we navigate the intricate landscape of implementing policies to combat PM2.5 pollution, challenges emerge as formidable obstacles on the journey towards cleaner air. Acknowledging these challenges is the first step towards devising effective strategies that can be tailored to the unique circumstances of each region. The chapters that follow will delve into specific case studies, success stories, and ongoing challenges related to government policies and regulations. The journey towards cleaner air involves not only understanding the complexities of implementation challenges but also forging a collective commitment to overcoming them for a healthier and sustainable future.

Policy Successes and Failures

As nations grapple with the formidable challenge of mitigating PM2.5 pollution, the effectiveness of government policies and regulations becomes a focal point of evaluation. This section explores both the successes and failures in the development and implementation of policies aimed at curbing the impacts of fine particulate matter. Understanding the intricacies of these outcomes is crucial for shaping future strategies and fostering a path toward cleaner air.

Success Stories: Pioneering Policies That Make a Difference

Stricter Emission Standards for Industries: One notable success in PM2.5 regulation is the implementation of stricter emission standards for industrial sources. Countries that have successfully enforced stringent limits on particulate matter emissions from power plants, manufacturing facilities, and other industrial processes have witnessed significant reductions in ambient PM2.5 concentrations. This success is often attributed to the adoption of advanced pollution control technologies and regular monitoring.

Transition to Cleaner Transportation: Policies promoting the transition to cleaner transportation have yielded positive outcomes in various regions. Countries that incentivize the use of electric vehicles, invest in public transportation infrastructure, and implement stringent vehicle emission standards have experienced improvements in air quality. The reduction of emissions from the transportation sector, a major contributor to PM2.5 pollution, contributes to healthier urban environments.

Integrated Urban Planning Initiatives: Success stories also emerge from cities that adopt integrated urban planning initiatives. Urban areas that prioritize green spaces, pedestrian-friendly infrastructure, and sustainable development have witnessed reductions in local PM2.5 concentrations. These initiatives not only contribute to improved air quality but also enhance overall urban livability.

Cross-Sectoral Collaboration: Policies that foster cross-sectoral collaboration have proven successful in addressing PM2.5 pollution comprehensively. Initiatives that bring together government agencies, industry stakeholders, environmental organizations, and the public contribute to a more holistic approach. Successful collaboration often leads to the development of integrated strategies that consider the diverse sources of fine particulate matter.

Analyzing Policy Failures: Unraveling Complex Challenges

Inadequate Enforcement Mechanisms: One significant failure in PM2.5 regulation often stems from inadequate enforcement mechanisms. Despite the existence of well-defined regulations, some regions struggle with enforcing compliance due to a lack of monitoring capabilities, insufficient staffing, and regulatory ambiguities. The failure to effectively enforce standards undermines the intended impact of policies.

Lack of Long-Term Planning: Policy failures also arise when there is a lack of long-term planning. In some cases, governments may implement short-term measures that address immediate concerns but fail to provide a sustainable framework for continuous improvement. Effective PM2.5 regulation requires a commitment to long-term planning that considers evolving environmental challenges and technological advancements.

Insufficient Public Awareness: Policies aimed at curbing PM2.5 pollution may falter when there is insufficient public awareness. In regions where the general population lacks understanding of the sources, health impacts, and mitigation measures related to fine particulate matter, policies may encounter resistance or apathy. Building public awareness is crucial for garnering support and fostering a sense of shared responsibility.

Policy Inconsistencies: Inconsistencies in environmental policies at different levels of government can impede effective regulation. When regional or municipal policies do not align with national standards, or when there are frequent changes in regulatory frameworks, industries may face challenges in compliance. Policy inconsistencies create uncertainty and hinder long-term planning.

Learning from Global Case Studies: Lessons in Effective Regulation

China's Air Pollution Action Plan: China's Air Pollution Action Plan, initiated in 2013, stands as a notable case of successful PM2.5 regulation. The plan included stringent emission standards for industries, increased monitoring capabilities, and a focus on transitioning to cleaner energy sources. As a result, major Chinese cities experienced notable reductions in PM2.5 concentrations, showcasing the impact of coordinated efforts on a national scale.

London's Congestion Charge: London's implementation of a congestion charge in the city center is a successful example of tackling PM2.5 pollution from transportation. By charging vehicles based on their emissions and encouraging the use of public transportation, London achieved a reduction in traffic-related air pollution. The success of this initiative highlights the effectiveness of targeted policies addressing specific pollution sources.

California's Zero-Emission Vehicle Mandate: California's Zero-Emission Vehicle (ZEV) mandate is a success story in promoting cleaner transportation. The state set ambitious targets for automakers to produce an increasing percentage of zero-emission vehicles. The mandate not only accelerated the adoption of electric vehicles but also contributed to a reduction in PM2.5 emissions from the transportation sector.

Paris Agreement's Co-Benefits: The Paris Agreement, while primarily focused on climate change, has demonstrated co-benefits in addressing air quality. Countries that align their climate action plans with air quality improvement goals contribute to a dual impact. This integration showcases the potential for global agreements to address interconnected environmental challenges.

Strategies for Future Success: A Blueprint for Effective Regulation

Strengthening Regulatory Enforcement: To overcome the challenge of inadequate enforcement, nations can focus on strengthening regulatory mechanisms. This includes investing in monitoring infrastructure, increasing staffing for regulatory agencies, and incorporating advanced technologies for real-time data collection. Clear communication and coordination among regulatory bodies are essential for effective enforcement.

Long-Term Planning and Adaptive Policies: Governments should prioritize long-term planning and develop adaptive policies that can evolve with changing circumstances. This involves considering future technological advancements, emerging sources of pollution, and potential shifts in economic priorities. Policies should be dynamic, allowing for adjustments based on ongoing monitoring and evaluation.

Public Awareness Campaigns: Addressing the issue of insufficient public awareness requires comprehensive public awareness campaigns. Governments can utilize various communication channels, including traditional media, social media, and community engagement initiatives, to educate the public about PM2.5 pollution, its sources, and the importance of individual and collective actions for cleaner air.

Harmonizing Policies Across Levels: Policy inconsistencies can be mitigated by harmonizing environmental policies across different levels of government. National standards should align with regional and local regulations to provide a cohesive framework for industries and communities.

Establishing mechanisms for ongoing collaboration and information exchange is essential.

Conclusion: Navigating the Road Ahead with Insights from the Past

As we navigate the complex landscape of PM2.5 regulation, the analysis of policy successes and failures provides invaluable insights. Learning from both positive outcomes and challenges is essential for shaping future strategies that can effectively address the impacts of fine particulate matter. The chapters that follow will delve deeper into specific case studies, emerging trends, and ongoing innovations in government policies and regulations, offering a comprehensive exploration of the multifaceted journey toward cleaner air.

Chapter 6: Technological Solutions

Innovative Technologies for PM2.5 Reduction

In the quest for cleaner air and the reduction of PM2.5 pollution, technological solutions play a pivotal role. This section explores a spectrum of innovative technologies designed to mitigate fine particulate matter emissions, highlighting breakthroughs that hold promise for a future where the air we breathe is healthier and safer for all.

1. Advanced Air Pollution Control Devices

Electrostatic Precipitators (ESPs): ESPs are electrostatic air cleaners that capture particulate matter through the use of an electric field. Charged particles adhere to collector plates, effectively removing them from the air. Modern ESPs are equipped with enhanced features such as high collection efficiency and low energy consumption, making them integral to industries seeking efficient particulate matter control.

Baghouses: Baghouses are filtration devices that use fabric bags to capture particles from gas streams. These bags, made from materials like felt or woven fabric, provide a large surface area for particle capture. Advances in baghouse technology include improved filtration materials, automated cleaning mechanisms, and modular designs that enhance efficiency and ease of maintenance.

Cyclone Separators: Cyclone separators use centrifugal force to separate particulate matter from air streams. These devices are effective for coarse particle removal and are often employed as pre-filters in air pollution control systems. Recent innovations include the development of high-efficiency cyclones with optimized geometries for enhanced particle collection.

2. Green Infrastructure and Urban Planning Innovations

Green Roofs and Walls: Integrating greenery into urban environments through green roofs and walls contributes to PM2.5 reduction. Plants act as natural filters, capturing particles from the air. Advances in green infrastructure include the development of specialized plant species that excel in air purification, as well as the integration of smart irrigation systems for optimized plant health.

Urban Forestry Strategies: Strategically planting and maintaining trees in urban areas can significantly reduce PM2.5 concentrations. Innovations in urban forestry include the use of data-driven approaches to identify optimal tree species and locations. Tree canopy mapping, coupled with air quality modeling, aids in designing urban landscapes that maximize the air purifying potential of trees.

Sustainable Urban Design: Holistic urban planning emphasizes sustainable design principles that consider air quality. Innovations include the development of pedestrian-friendly zones, efficient public transportation systems, and mixed-use urban spaces that reduce reliance on individual vehicles. These approaches not only enhance overall urban livability but also contribute to lower PM2.5 levels.

3. Clean Energy Solutions

Solar Air Purifiers: Solar-powered air purifiers utilize photovoltaic cells to generate energy for air purification processes. These devices can be deployed in urban areas and industrial zones, using solar energy to power air filtration systems. Solar air purifiers represent a sustainable solution, especially in regions with abundant sunlight, addressing both energy consumption and air quality challenges.

Renewable Energy Integration: Transitioning to renewable energy sources, such as wind and solar power, contributes to PM2.5 reduction by decreasing emissions from fossil fuel combustion. Innovations in renewable energy technologies, including advanced wind turbine designs and efficient solar panels, play a crucial role in creating a cleaner energy landscape with positive implications for air quality.

Electric Vehicles and Transportation Electrification: The electrification of transportation, particularly the widespread adoption of electric vehicles (EVs), reduces emissions from traditional internal combustion engines. Innovations in EV technology include advancements in battery efficiency, fast-charging infrastructure, and the integration of renewable energy sources into charging networks.

4. Smart Technologies and Monitoring Systems

Low-Cost Air Quality Sensors: Low-cost air quality sensors enable real-time monitoring of PM2.5 concentrations at a granular level. These sensors, often connected to digital platforms, empower individuals and communities to track air quality in their surroundings. Ongoing innovations focus on improving sensor accuracy, data reliability, and the integration of sensor networks for comprehensive coverage.

Satellite-Based Monitoring: Satellite technology offers a broader perspective on air quality by providing global-scale monitoring. Satellites equipped with remote sensing instruments can capture data on aerosol concentrations, allowing for the observation of regional and transboundary PM2.5 patterns. Advances in satellite-based monitoring contribute to a more comprehensive understanding of air quality dynamics.

Data Analytics and Artificial Intelligence: Data analytics and artificial intelligence (AI) play a crucial role in processing large volumes of air quality data. AI algorithms can analyze complex datasets to identify patterns, predict pollution events, and optimize the operation of pollution control systems. Innovations in AI applications for air quality management enhance decision-making and response strategies.

5. Industrial Process Optimization

Cleaner Manufacturing Processes: Innovations in industrial processes aim to reduce particulate matter emissions at the source. Advanced manufacturing technologies, such as 3D printing and precision machining, minimize the generation of fine particles during production. Additionally, sustainable practices, including closed-loop manufacturing and circular economy principles, contribute to cleaner industrial operations.

Carbon Capture and Utilization (CCU): CCU technologies capture carbon dioxide emissions from industrial processes and convert them into valuable products. By addressing multiple pollutants, including particulate matter, CCU contributes to comprehensive air quality improvement. Ongoing innovations focus on optimizing CCU processes and exploring novel applications for captured carbon.

Emission Reduction Technologies: Industries are adopting innovative emission reduction technologies, such as catalytic converters and flue gas desulfurization systems, to minimize the release of pollutants, including PM2.5. Advances in these technologies include the development of catalyst materials with enhanced efficiency and the integration of real-time monitoring for adaptive control.

6. Collaborative Research and Cross-Sectoral Solutions

Public-Private Partnerships: Collaborative initiatives between government agencies, private industries, research institutions, and non-governmental organizations play a crucial role in developing and implementing innovative PM2.5 reduction technologies. Public-private partnerships foster the exchange of knowledge, resources, and expertise, accelerating the translation of research findings into practical solutions.

Cross-Sectoral Integration: Addressing PM2.5 pollution requires a cross-sectoral approach that integrates solutions from diverse fields. Innovations emerge when industries, environmental scientists, urban planners, and policymakers collaborate to develop comprehensive strategies. Cross-sectoral integration facilitates the identification of synergies and the creation of holistic solutions that consider the interconnected nature of air quality challenges.

Global Research Networks: Global research networks and collaborative projects contribute to the development of cutting-edge technologies for PM2.5 reduction. International collaboration fosters the sharing of best practices, facilitates joint research initiatives, and accelerates the dissemination of technological innovations. Participating in global research networks enhances the collective capacity to address air quality challenges.

Conclusion: Embracing a Technological Revolution for Cleaner Air

As we delve into the realm of innovative technologies for PM2.5 reduction, a technological revolution unfolds, offering a glimpse into a future where cleaner air is not only a possibility but a tangible reality. The chapters that follow will explore specific case studies, success stories, and ongoing challenges related to the implementation and advancement of technological solutions in the global pursuit of healthier air quality.

Clean Energy Initiatives

In the relentless pursuit of cleaner air, clean energy initiatives emerge as a transformative force, offering innovative solutions to combat PM2.5 pollution. This section explores a spectrum of clean energy technologies and initiatives that not only reduce particulate matter emissions but also pave the way for sustainable and resilient energy landscapes.

Transitioning to Renewable Energy Sources

Solar Power Revolution: Solar energy stands at the forefront of the clean energy revolution, presenting a sustainable alternative to traditional fossil fuels. Photovoltaic (PV) solar panels convert sunlight into electricity, eliminating the combustion of fossil fuels that releases PM2.5 and other pollutants. Innovations in solar technology include advancements in panel efficiency, storage solutions, and the integration of solar farms into urban landscapes.

Wind Energy Advancements: Harnessing the power of the wind has become a key strategy for reducing reliance on polluting energy sources. Wind turbines generate electricity without emitting particulate matter, contributing to cleaner air. Technological advancements in wind energy include the development of larger and more efficient turbines, offshore wind farms, and smart grid integration for enhanced reliability.

Hydropower Innovations: Hydropower, derived from the energy of flowing water, provides a clean and renewable energy source. Unlike traditional power generation methods, hydropower does not release particulate matter during electricity generation. Innovations in hydropower technology include run-of-river systems, tidal energy capture, and fish-friendly turbine designs that minimize environmental impact.

Electrification of Transportation

Electric Vehicles (EVs): The electrification of transportation represents a pivotal clean energy initiative, addressing PM2.5 pollution from the combustion of fossil fuels in internal combustion engines. Electric vehicles, powered by batteries or fuel cells, produce zero tailpipe emissions, significantly reducing particulate matter released into the air. Innovations in EV technology focus on increasing battery efficiency, extending range, and enhancing charging infrastructure.

Public Transportation Electrification: Beyond individual vehicles, the electrification of public transportation systems plays a crucial role in reducing emissions from buses, trains, and trams. Electric buses, for example, offer a cleaner alternative to traditional diesel-powered counterparts. Innovations in public transportation electrification include rapid charging stations, battery swapping technologies, and the integration of renewable energy sources into transit networks.

Alternative Fuels and Sustainable Mobility: Clean energy initiatives extend to alternative fuels such as hydrogen and biofuels, providing options for reducing PM2.5 emissions in transportation. Sustainable mobility solutions include the development of hydrogen fuel cell vehicles, the use of biofuels derived from renewable sources, and the implementation of smart transportation systems to optimize traffic flow and reduce congestion.

Decentralized and Off-Grid Solutions

Solar Microgrids: Decentralized energy systems, particularly solar microgrids, offer clean energy solutions in areas where centralized power infrastructure is limited. These microgrids harness solar energy to provide electricity to communities, reducing reliance on diesel generators and other sources associated with PM2.5 emissions. Innovations include energy storage technologies for continuous power supply and the integration of microgrid systems into rural and remote areas.

Biomass Gasification: Biomass gasification technology converts organic waste into clean energy, reducing reliance on traditional biomass burning practices that release particulate matter. Innovations in biomass gasification include improved gasifier designs, efficient energy conversion processes, and the utilization of agricultural residues, wood waste, or organic municipal solid waste as feedstocks.

Off-Grid Renewable Solutions: Clean energy initiatives extend to off-grid applications, such as standalone solar systems and small-scale wind turbines. These solutions provide reliable and sustainable power in remote locations, reducing the need for diesel generators that contribute to PM2.5 pollution. Innovations focus on enhancing the efficiency and affordability of off-grid renewable technologies.

Integration of Smart Technologies

Smart Grids for Energy Optimization: Smart grids represent a technological leap in optimizing energy distribution and consumption. These systems leverage advanced sensors, communication networks, and data analytics to enhance the efficiency of energy grids. By reducing energy wastage and promoting load balancing, smart grids contribute to a cleaner energy landscape, minimizing the environmental footprint associated with power generation.

Energy Storage Solutions: The integration of energy storage solutions, such as advanced batteries and flywheel systems, plays a pivotal role in clean energy initiatives. Storage technologies enable the efficient use of renewable energy by storing excess power generated during periods of high production for use during low-production periods. Innovations in energy storage focus on increasing capacity, lifespan, and recyclability.

Demand Response Systems: Demand response systems utilize smart technologies to manage energy consumption in real-time, aligning it with the availability of renewable energy. By incentivizing consumers to adjust their energy usage based on grid conditions, these systems contribute to a more flexible and sustainable energy grid. Innovations include the integration of artificial intelligence for predictive demand modeling and automated response mechanisms.

Government Policies and Incentives

Renewable Energy Targets: Governments worldwide are setting ambitious renewable energy targets to transition away from fossil fuels. These targets often include specific goals for solar, wind, hydropower, and other clean energy sources. Innovations in policy frameworks include the establishment of feed-in tariffs, tax incentives, and regulatory mechanisms that encourage investment in clean energy projects.

Green Energy Certification Programs: Certification programs, such as Green Power Certification, verify and promote the use of clean energy sources. These programs provide consumers, businesses, and governments with transparent information about the environmental attributes of their energy sources. Innovations include the development of blockchain-based certification systems for increased transparency and traceability.

Carbon Pricing Initiatives: Carbon pricing mechanisms, including carbon taxes and cap-and-trade systems, incentivize the reduction of greenhouse gas emissions, including those associated with PM2.5 pollution. These initiatives create economic incentives for industries to transition to cleaner energy sources and implement pollution control measures. Innovations in carbon pricing include international collaborations to establish consistent and effective pricing mechanisms.

Global Collaborations and Research Initiatives

International Research Collaborations: Clean energy initiatives benefit from global collaborations that foster the exchange of knowledge, expertise, and research findings. International research networks focus on developing cutting-edge technologies, sharing best practices, and addressing common challenges associated with the transition to clean energy. Innovations emerge through joint projects that leverage diverse perspectives and resources.

Technology Transfer Programs: Technology transfer programs facilitate the dissemination of clean energy innovations from developed to developing nations. These programs aim to bridge the technology gap and accelerate the adoption of clean energy solutions in regions facing energy access challenges. Innovations in technology transfer include capacity-building initiatives and partnerships between research institutions, governments, and industries.

Global Renewable Energy Partnerships: Global partnerships dedicated to renewable energy promote collaborative efforts in advancing clean energy solutions. These partnerships involve governments, businesses, and non-governmental organizations working together to accelerate the deployment of renewable energy technologies. Innovations in global renewable energy collaborations include funding mechanisms, knowledge-sharing platforms, and joint initiatives for sustainable development.

Conclusion: Catalyzing Change Through Clean Energy Innovations

As we explore the realm of clean energy initiatives, a profound transformation unfolds—a transformation that not only reduces PM2.5 pollution but also charts a course towards a sustainable and resilient energy future. The chapters that follow will delve into specific case studies, success stories, and ongoing challenges related to clean energy technologies, offering a comprehensive exploration of the role of innovative solutions in shaping a cleaner and healthier environment.

Air Quality Monitoring Advancements

In the dynamic landscape of combating PM2.5 pollution, the role of advanced air quality monitoring technologies cannot be overstated. This section explores the latest innovations and advancements in air quality monitoring, offering a comprehensive view of the tools and techniques that empower individuals, communities, and governments to take proactive measures in the pursuit of cleaner air.

1. Low-Cost Air Quality Sensors: Pioneering Accessibility

Overview of Low-Cost Sensors: Low-cost air quality sensors have emerged as game-changers in the realm of air quality monitoring. These compact devices, often affordable and portable, enable individuals and communities to measure particulate matter concentrations in real-time. Innovations in low-cost sensor technology include enhanced accuracy, reduced power consumption, and the integration of wireless connectivity for seamless data transmission.

Community-Led Monitoring Initiatives: The rise of low-cost sensors has sparked community-led monitoring initiatives, empowering citizens to actively participate in assessing and addressing local air quality issues. Community networks equipped with these sensors provide real-time data, creating a more granular understanding of PM2.5 concentrations in specific neighborhoods. Innovations in community-led monitoring include the development of user-friendly interfaces and participatory data interpretation platforms.

Challenges and Calibration Strategies: While low-cost sensors offer increased accessibility, challenges such as calibration and data accuracy persist. Ongoing innovations focus on developing robust calibration methods, including sensor calibration stations and machine learning algorithms that adjust for sensor drift over time. Calibration strategies play a crucial role in ensuring the reliability of data collected by low-cost sensors.

2. Satellite-Based Monitoring: A Global Perspective

Advancements in Satellite Technology: Satellite-based monitoring provides a global perspective on air quality, offering insights into regional and transboundary PM2.5 patterns. Modern satellites equipped with advanced remote sensing instruments capture detailed data on aerosol concentrations, contributing to a comprehensive understanding of air quality dynamics. Innovations include improved spatial and temporal resolution, allowing for more detailed observations.

Integration with Ground-Based Data: Combining satellite observations with ground-based data enhances the accuracy and reliability of air quality monitoring. Integrated systems leverage the strengths of both satellite and ground-based technologies to create a holistic view of PM2.5 concentrations. Innovations in data fusion techniques and machine learning algorithms enable seamless integration, providing policymakers with a more comprehensive toolkit for decision-making.

Global Collaborations for Data Sharing: Satellite-based monitoring benefits from global collaborations that facilitate data sharing and harmonization. International efforts involve the establishment of data-sharing agreements, standardized data formats, and collaborative research initiatives. Innovations in global data-sharing platforms contribute to a more interconnected and accessible repository of satellite-derived air quality data.

3. Artificial Intelligence and Data Analytics: Unleashing Insights

Role of Artificial Intelligence (AI): The integration of AI and data analytics revolutionizes the analysis of air quality data, uncovering patterns and trends that may elude traditional methods. AI algorithms process vast datasets to identify correlations, predict pollution events, and optimize the operation of pollution control systems. Innovations include machine learning models capable of real-time data interpretation and adaptive decision-making.

Smart Sensor Networks: The deployment of smart sensor networks, equipped with AI capabilities, enhances the efficiency of air quality monitoring. These networks consist of interconnected sensors that communicate and share data in real-time. Innovations in smart sensor networks include self-calibrating sensors, adaptive sampling strategies, and the use of edge computing for on-device data processing.

Predictive Modeling for PM2.5: Predictive modeling powered by AI allows for forecasting PM2.5 concentrations based on historical data, meteorological factors, and other relevant variables. These models enable proactive measures to mitigate pollution events and inform public health interventions. Innovations in predictive modeling include the incorporation of real-time data feeds, ensemble modeling approaches, and continuous model refinement.

4. Continuous Emission Monitoring Systems: Industry Accountability

Introduction to Continuous Emission Monitoring Systems (CEMS): CEMS are vital tools for industries to monitor and report their emissions, including particulate matter. These systems provide real-time data on pollutant releases, enabling industries to track compliance with regulatory standards and implement timely corrective measures. Innovations in CEMS include the integration of advanced sensors, data connectivity, and remote monitoring capabilities.

Real-Time Compliance Monitoring: CEMS contribute to real-time compliance monitoring by providing instant feedback on emission levels. Innovations in this area focus on automating compliance reporting, leveraging cloud-based platforms for data storage and analysis, and integrating CEMS with regulatory frameworks for streamlined reporting processes.

Remote Monitoring for Remote Industries: Remote industries, often located in challenging terrains, benefit from the remote monitoring capabilities of CEMS. Innovations include the use of satellite communication, IoT-enabled sensors, and ruggedized monitoring equipment that withstands harsh environmental conditions. These advancements ensure that even industries in remote locations can contribute to the reduction of PM2.5 emissions.

5. Drones and Mobile Monitoring Platforms: Dynamic Data Collection

Role of Drones in Air Quality Monitoring: Drones, equipped with air quality sensors, offer a dynamic and flexible approach to data collection. These aerial platforms can access hard-to-reach or hazardous areas, providing a comprehensive view of PM2.5 concentrations. Innovations in drone-based monitoring include the development of autonomous flight paths, real-time data transmission, and the integration of multiple sensors for simultaneous pollutant detection.

Mobile Monitoring Units: Mobile monitoring units, mounted on vehicles or carried by pedestrians, bring air quality monitoring to different locations and scenarios. These units enable the mapping of PM2.5 concentrations across diverse environments, offering valuable insights for urban planning and pollution mitigation strategies. Innovations in mobile monitoring platforms include lightweight and compact sensors, advanced data visualization tools, and real-time mapping capabilities.

Crowdsourced Data Collection Initiatives: The use of mobile apps and crowdsourced data collection initiatives engages citizens in monitoring air quality on the go. Individuals equipped with smartphones can contribute real-time data, creating a dynamic and continuously updated air quality map. Innovations include gamified apps, community challenges, and the integration of crowdsourced data into official monitoring systems.

6. Integration with Health Data: Bridging the Gap

Health Data Integration for Holistic Insights: The integration of air quality data with health data creates a more holistic understanding of the impact of PM2.5 pollution on public health. Combining information on respiratory conditions, hospital admissions, and epidemiological trends allows for a comprehensive assessment of the health consequences of air pollution. Innovations include health data analytics platforms that correlate air quality indicators with health outcomes.

Real-Time Health Alerts: Advanced air quality monitoring systems, integrated with health databases, can generate real-time health alerts. These alerts inform the public, healthcare professionals, and policymakers about potential health risks associated with elevated PM2.5 levels. Innovations in real-time health alerts include automated messaging systems, mobile app notifications, and web-based platforms for dissemination.

Longitudinal Health Studies: Longitudinal studies that track the health of populations over time provide valuable insights into the chronic effects of PM2.5 exposure. Integrating air quality data into these studies contributes to a deeper understanding of the long-term health consequences of air pollution. Innovations include collaborative research frameworks that bring together environmental scientists, epidemiologists, and healthcare professionals.

Conclusion: Shaping a Future of Informed Action

As we navigate the landscape of air quality monitoring advancements, a future of informed action and empowered communities comes into focus. The chapters that follow will delve into specific case studies, success stories, and ongoing challenges related to the implementation and advancement of air quality monitoring technologies. These innovations serve as catalysts for change, fostering a world where individuals and societies can actively participate in the collective effort to combat PM2.5 pollution.

Role of Data and Technology in Mitigation

In the ongoing battle against PM2.5 pollution, the convergence of data and technology emerges as a powerful force, providing the tools needed to understand, monitor, and mitigate the impact of fine particulate matter on air quality. This section explores the pivotal role played by data-driven technologies in shaping effective strategies for mitigating PM2.5 pollution and fostering a future of cleaner air.

Harnessing Big Data for Precision Insights

Overview of Big Data in Air Quality Management: Big data analytics revolutionizes the field of air quality management, offering unprecedented insights into the sources, dispersion, and impact of PM2.5 pollution. The sheer volume and variety of data generated from air quality sensors, satellite observations, and other monitoring platforms provide a rich foundation for understanding the dynamics of particulate matter in the atmosphere.

Real-Time Monitoring and Decision-Making: Big data enables real-time monitoring of PM2.5 concentrations, facilitating timely decision-making by governments, industries, and individuals. Advanced analytics platforms process vast datasets to detect pollution events, predict trends, and optimize the deployment of pollution control measures. Innovations in real-time data analytics include the use of machine learning algorithms for rapid pattern recognition and anomaly detection.

Data Fusion for Comprehensive Understanding: Integrating data from various sources, including ground-based sensors, satellite observations, and meteorological data, creates a comprehensive understanding of PM2.5 dynamics. Data fusion techniques enhance the accuracy and reliability of air quality assessments, providing a more nuanced view of pollution sources and dispersion patterns. Innovations include automated data fusion algorithms that adapt to changing conditions and evolving sensor technologies.

Citizen Science and Participatory Monitoring

Empowering Communities Through Data: Citizen science initiatives leverage technology to empower communities in monitoring and mitigating PM2.5 pollution. Mobile apps, low-cost sensors, and online platforms enable citizens to actively contribute to air quality data collection. Innovations in citizen science include gamified apps that encourage engagement, community-led monitoring networks, and participatory mapping tools that visualize local air quality data.

Enhancing Public Awareness and Advocacy: Data generated through citizen science initiatives not only contributes to scientific understanding but also enhances public awareness of air quality issues. Communities armed with actionable data become advocates for cleaner air, pressuring authorities to implement effective mitigation strategies. Innovations in public engagement include social media campaigns, interactive data visualization tools, and community forums for sharing insights and experiences.

Integration with Official Monitoring Systems: Citizen-generated data can complement and enrich official air quality monitoring systems. Collaborative efforts between citizens and government agencies foster a more inclusive and transparent approach to air quality management. Innovations include standardized data formats, interoperable sensor networks, and mechanisms for integrating citizen-generated data into regulatory frameworks.

Smart Cities and Urban Planning Solutions

Smart Cities as Laboratories for Air Quality Innovation: Smart cities leverage technology to create sustainable and livable urban environments. Integrated sensor networks, smart infrastructure, and data analytics platforms contribute to effective air quality management. Innovations in smart cities include the deployment of sensors in public spaces, smart transportation systems that reduce traffic-related emissions, and urban planning strategies that prioritize air quality.

Data-Driven Urban Planning: The integration of air quality data into urban planning processes enables the development of strategies to mitigate PM2.5 pollution. Data-driven urban planning considers factors such as green spaces, traffic management, and industrial zoning to create environments that support cleaner air. Innovations include the use of geospatial analytics, predictive modeling, and real-time data feeds to inform urban development decisions.

Sustainable Mobility Solutions: Smart cities embrace sustainable mobility solutions that reduce emissions from transportation, a significant contributor to PM2.5 pollution. Technologies such as intelligent traffic management systems, electric public transportation, and bike-sharing programs contribute to cleaner urban air. Innovations in sustainable mobility include the integration of real-time air quality data into navigation apps, incentivizing eco-friendly transportation choices.

Industrial Process Optimization

Smart Manufacturing for Emission Reduction: Industries are adopting smart manufacturing technologies to optimize processes and reduce emissions, including particulate matter. Internet of Things (IoT) devices, real-time monitoring systems, and data analytics enable industries to identify opportunities for emission reduction. Innovations include smart sensors that monitor equipment performance, predictive maintenance algorithms, and cloud-based platforms for remote monitoring.

Emission Control Technologies: Advanced emission control technologies play a crucial role in mitigating PM2.5 pollution from industrial sources. Technologies such as electrostatic precipitators, baghouses, and catalytic converters are integrated into industrial processes to capture and reduce particulate matter emissions. Innovations in emission control include the development of high-efficiency filters, continuous monitoring systems, and closed-loop manufacturing processes.

Data-Driven Compliance Monitoring: Data analytics platforms are employed for continuous compliance monitoring in industries. Real-time data analysis ensures that industrial processes adhere to regulatory standards, minimizing the release of particulate matter into the air. Innovations include automated reporting systems, machine learning algorithms for anomaly detection, and cloud-based compliance platforms that enhance transparency.

International Collaboration and Knowledge Sharing

Global Data Platforms for Air Quality: International collaboration is facilitated by global data platforms that provide a shared repository of air quality data. These platforms enable countries to compare, analyze, and learn from each other's experiences in mitigating PM2.5 pollution. Innovations include standardized data formats, open-access databases, and collaborative research initiatives that contribute to a collective understanding of air quality challenges.

Joint Research Initiatives for Technological Solutions: Collaborative research initiatives bring together experts from different countries to work on technological solutions for PM2.5 mitigation. Joint projects focus on developing and testing innovations in air quality monitoring, emission reduction technologies, and data analytics. Innovations include research networks, joint funding mechanisms, and technology transfer programs that accelerate the adoption of effective solutions.

Capacity Building and Technical Assistance: International collaborations prioritize capacity building and technical assistance to support countries in their efforts to mitigate PM2.5 pollution. Training programs, knowledge exchange forums, and mentorship initiatives contribute to the development of expertise in air quality management. Innovations include virtual training platforms, cross-border knowledge-sharing events, and partnerships between research institutions and government agencies.

Conclusion: A Data-Driven Future for Clean Air

As we explore the intricate interplay of data and technology in the mitigation of PM2.5 pollution, a future emerges where informed decision-making, community engagement, and international collaboration become the cornerstones of cleaner air. The chapters that follow will delve into specific case studies, success stories, and ongoing challenges related to the implementation and advancement of data-driven technologies in the fight against PM2.5 pollution. These innovations not only shape the present but pave the way for a future where the air we breathe is a testament to the transformative power of data and technology.

Chapter 7: Public Awareness and Advocacy

Public Perception of Air Quality

The perception of air quality is a dynamic interplay between individual experiences, community awareness, and broader societal narratives. Understanding how the public perceives air quality is crucial for effective advocacy and mobilization efforts. This section explores the various dimensions of public perception, shedding light on the factors influencing awareness, concerns, and the potential for collective action in the face of PM2.5 pollution.

Perception and Reality: Bridging the Gap

The Invisible Threat: PM2.5 and Its Elusive Nature: Particulate matter, especially PM2.5, is often referred to as the invisible enemy. Its microscopic size renders it imperceptible to the human eye, creating a challenge in conveying its presence and impact. Public perception is influenced by the difficulty in visualizing these tiny particles, leading to a potential gap between the reality of air quality and the public's understanding.

Educational Initiatives and Awareness Campaigns: Bridging the gap between perception and reality requires targeted educational initiatives and awareness campaigns. Efforts to explain the science behind PM2.5, its sources, and health implications play a pivotal role in shaping public understanding. Innovations in communication include the use of multimedia resources, interactive platforms, and community-based workshops to make complex information accessible and engaging.

Media Representation and Framing: Media plays a significant role in shaping public perception of air quality. The way in which air quality issues are framed in news stories, documentaries, and social media platforms influences how the public interprets and reacts to information. Innovations in media representation include data visualization tools, real-time air quality reporting, and storytelling approaches that humanize the impact of PM2.5 pollution on individuals and communities.

Factors Influencing Public Perception

Sensory Experience and Immediate Impacts: Public perception is often shaped by sensory experiences and immediate impacts on health. Individuals may become more aware of air quality issues when they directly experience symptoms such as respiratory irritation or notice visible signs like smog. Innovations in personal air quality monitoring devices and health tracking apps empower individuals to connect their daily experiences with broader air quality concerns.

Geographical and Temporal Variability: The perception of air quality is influenced by geographical and temporal variability. Residents of areas with chronic air quality issues may develop heightened awareness, while those in regions with generally good air quality may be less attuned to the issue. Innovations include real-time air quality maps, localized reporting, and community-based monitoring programs that provide context-specific information.

Community Engagement and Social Networks: Social dynamics play a crucial role in shaping public perception. Community engagement and discussions within social networks contribute to the spread of information and the formation of shared beliefs. Innovations in community engagement include online forums, social media campaigns, and community-led air quality monitoring initiatives that foster a sense of shared responsibility and concern.

Public Awareness Campaigns and Behavioral Change

The Power of Public Awareness Campaigns: Public awareness campaigns serve as catalysts for shaping perception and promoting behavioral change. These campaigns leverage various mediums, including television, radio, online platforms, and community events, to disseminate information about the impact of PM2.5 pollution and encourage sustainable practices. Innovations in awareness campaigns include gamification, augmented reality experiences, and collaborations with influencers to reach diverse audiences.

Behavioral Nudges for Cleaner Air Practices: Public perception is intimately linked to individual behaviors. Behavioral nudges, informed by behavioral economics and psychology, aim to subtly guide individuals toward making choices that contribute to cleaner air. Innovations in behavioral nudges include personalized air quality alerts, eco-feedback apps, and incentive-based programs that reward individuals for adopting sustainable practices.

Incorporating Air Quality in Educational Curricula: Educational institutions play a vital role in shaping the attitudes and awareness of future generations. Integrating air quality education into school curricula provides a foundation for understanding environmental issues and fosters a sense of responsibility. Innovations in educational approaches include interactive digital resources, virtual reality simulations, and outdoor learning experiences that connect students with real-world air quality challenges.

Challenges in Public Awareness

Misinformation and Lack of Understanding: The prevalence of misinformation and a lack of understanding about air quality issues pose challenges to public awareness efforts. Addressing these challenges requires targeted communication strategies that debunk myths, provide accurate information, and clarify the sources and consequences of PM2.5 pollution. Innovations include fact-checking tools, online platforms for expert Q&A sessions, and collaborative initiatives with influencers to counter misinformation.

Complacency in Regions with Moderate Air Quality: In regions where air quality is moderate or considered acceptable by regulatory standards, there may be a sense of complacency among the public. Overcoming this complacency involves highlighting the long-term health impacts of even moderate exposure to PM2.5 and emphasizing the benefits of sustained efforts toward cleaner air. Innovations include personalized health risk assessments, citizen science projects, and storytelling campaigns that resonate with diverse communities.

Limited Access to Information in Vulnerable Communities: Vulnerable communities, often disproportionately affected by air pollution, may face barriers to accessing information and resources. Overcoming this challenge requires targeted outreach efforts, community-driven initiatives, and partnerships with local organizations. Innovations in outreach include multilingual communication, mobile-friendly information platforms, and community-based participatory research projects that prioritize the needs of vulnerable populations.

Opportunities for Advocacy and Mobilization

Digital Platforms for Grassroots Advocacy: The rise of digital platforms provides opportunities for grassroots advocacy and mobilization. Online campaigns, petitions, and social media movements amplify the voices of individuals advocating for cleaner air. Innovations in digital advocacy include crowdfunding initiatives, virtual events, and collaborative platforms that connect activists, experts, and concerned citizens across geographical boundaries.

Citizen Science as a Catalyst for Change: Citizen science initiatives empower individuals to actively contribute to air quality monitoring and advocacy. Engaging citizens as active participants in data collection and analysis fosters a sense of ownership and agency. Innovations in citizen science include mobile apps for data collection, community-driven research projects, and partnerships between citizen scientists and academic institutions.

Inclusive and Culturally Relevant Messaging: Culturally relevant messaging that resonates with diverse communities is essential for effective advocacy. Recognizing the cultural, social, and economic factors that shape public perception allows advocates to tailor their messaging to specific audiences. Innovations in inclusive messaging include collaborations with cultural influencers, multilingual communication strategies, and storytelling that reflects the lived experiences of different communities.

Conclusion: Nurturing Informed Advocacy

As we navigate the complex terrain of public perception of air quality, it becomes evident that informed advocacy is nurtured through a combination of education, engagement, and targeted communication. The chapters that follow will delve into specific case studies, successful advocacy campaigns, and ongoing challenges related to shaping public awareness and mobilizing communities in the fight against PM2.5 pollution. These innovations not only amplify the urgency of the issue but also inspire collective action for a future where clean air is a shared priority.

Community Initiatives

At the heart of the battle against PM2.5 pollution lies the power of communities to initiate change. This section explores the diverse range of community initiatives aimed at raising awareness, fostering collaboration, and advocating for cleaner air. From neighborhood-led monitoring projects to innovative grassroots campaigns, these initiatives showcase the potency of community-driven efforts in the fight against particulate matter pollution.

Empowering Communities Through Monitoring

Community-Led Air Quality Monitoring Networks: In many regions, communities have taken the lead in monitoring their own air quality. Community-led networks deploy low-cost sensors and engage residents in collecting real-time data, providing a localized understanding of PM2.5 levels. These initiatives empower communities to actively participate in the monitoring process, fostering a sense of ownership and accountability.

Citizen Science Projects for Data Collection: Citizen science projects leverage the collective power of community members to contribute valuable data on air quality. Engaging citizens in scientific processes, these initiatives often include hands-on training, workshops, and collaborative data collection efforts. Community members become citizen scientists, bridging the gap between expert knowledge and local insights.

Interactive Mapping Platforms: Interactive mapping platforms provide communities with accessible tools to visualize and share air quality data. These platforms allow residents to map pollution hotspots, track trends, and collaboratively address local challenges. Community members can use the maps for advocacy, influencing local policies, and fostering a greater sense of environmental stewardship.

Education and Awareness Initiatives

Environmental Education Programs: Schools and community centers play a crucial role in educating the next generation about air quality issues. Environmental education programs integrate lessons on PM2.5 pollution, its sources, and the importance of clean air practices. These initiatives instill a sense of environmental responsibility in young minds, fostering a generation that is informed and proactive.

Workshops and Seminars: Community-led workshops and seminars bring together residents, experts, and local authorities to discuss air quality concerns. These interactive sessions delve into the science behind PM2.5 pollution, its health implications, and strategies for mitigation. Workshops serve as platforms for knowledge exchange, empowering communities with the information needed to make informed decisions.

Community Health Screenings: Some community initiatives go beyond education to directly address the health impacts of PM2.5 pollution. Collaborating with healthcare professionals, communities organize health screenings to assess the impact of air quality on residents' well-being. These screenings create a tangible link between air quality and health outcomes, motivating communities to advocate for cleaner air.

Advocacy and Community Engagement

Community-Based Advocacy Campaigns: Grassroots advocacy campaigns mobilize community members to advocate for policies that address PM2.5 pollution. These campaigns often involve door-to-door outreach, community meetings, and the use of traditional and digital media to amplify messages. Grassroots advocates leverage community voices to influence decision-makers at the local and regional levels.

Art and Culture for Advocacy: Art and cultural initiatives serve as powerful tools for community advocacy. Murals, performances, and installations centered around air quality draw attention to the issue in a creative and engaging manner. Artistic expressions not only convey the urgency of the problem but also inspire collective action and a shared commitment to cleaner air.

Community-Based Policy Dialogues: Engaging communities in policy dialogues ensures that their voices are heard in decision-making processes. Community leaders, residents, and experts participate in dialogues with policymakers to discuss the specific challenges and solutions related to PM2.5 pollution. These initiatives create a platform for inclusive decision-making and foster a sense of shared responsibility.

Innovative Community-Led Campaigns

Community Challenges and Competitions: Community challenges and competitions gamify the process of advocating for clean air. Whether it's a friendly competition to reduce individual carbon footprints or a community challenge to plant trees, these initiatives make environmental stewardship accessible and enjoyable. Incentives, such as prizes or community recognition, further motivate participation.

Tech-Savvy Community Apps: In the digital age, communities are leveraging technology to connect and collaborate. Community apps dedicated to air quality allow residents to report pollution incidents, share insights, and access real-time data. These apps foster a sense of community engagement, enabling residents to stay informed and actively contribute to local air quality improvements.

Community-Led Green Initiatives: Green initiatives led by communities involve activities like tree planting, community gardens, and sustainable waste management projects. These initiatives not only contribute to environmental conservation but also enhance community resilience against the impacts of PM2.5 pollution. Green spaces act as natural filters, improving local air quality and fostering a sense of communal well-being.

Challenges and Opportunities for Community Initiatives

Resource Limitations in Underserved Communities: Underserved communities may face resource limitations in implementing air quality initiatives. Lack of funding, access to technology, and educational resources can hinder community-led efforts. Addressing these challenges requires targeted support, partnerships with organizations, and advocacy for equitable distribution of resources.

Cultural and Linguistic Diversity: Cultural and linguistic diversity poses both challenges and opportunities for community initiatives. Tailoring campaigns to resonate with diverse cultural backgrounds is essential for effective communication. Embracing cultural diversity allows for creative and inclusive approaches that amplify the impact of community-driven initiatives.

Scaling Up Successful Community Models: Successful community initiatives often face the challenge of scaling up their impact. Identifying and replicating successful models in other communities require strategic planning, knowledge exchange platforms, and support from local governments and environmental organizations. Scaling up ensures that effective community-driven approaches can create a ripple effect in addressing PM2.5 pollution.

Conclusion: The Power of Collective Action

As we explore the myriad ways in which communities are taking the lead in combating PM2.5 pollution, the resounding theme is the power of collective action. The chapters that follow will delve into specific case studies, lessons learned from successful community initiatives, and ongoing challenges related to community-led efforts. These innovations not only empower communities but also underscore the transformative potential of grassroots movements in the pursuit of cleaner air.

Advocacy Campaigns and Movements

Advocacy campaigns and movements dedicated to addressing PM2.5 pollution play a pivotal role in mobilizing public sentiment, influencing policy changes, and fostering a collective commitment to cleaner air. This section explores the diverse landscape of advocacy campaigns and movements, from global initiatives to locally-driven efforts, showcasing the transformative power of strategic communication, grassroots organizing, and public mobilization.

Global Advocacy Initiatives

The BreatheLife Campaign: Launched by the World Health Organization (WHO), the United Nations Environment Programme (UNEP), and the Climate & Clean Air Coalition (CCAC), the BreatheLife campaign aims to mobilize cities and individuals to take action against air pollution. Through a combination of advocacy, awareness-building, and collaboration with cities worldwide, the campaign encourages the adoption of clean air policies and practices.

Clean Air Asia's Initiatives: Clean Air Asia, a regional network that works towards better air quality management in Asia, leads multiple advocacy initiatives. Their campaigns focus on promoting sustainable transportation, enhancing awareness about air quality issues, and engaging with policymakers to implement effective measures. Clean Air Asia's efforts highlight the importance of regional collaboration in addressing air pollution challenges.

The Climate Reality Project: Founded by former U.S. Vice President Al Gore, The Climate Reality Project is a global organization dedicated to mobilizing action on climate change, including air quality issues. Their advocacy efforts involve training activists, conducting awareness campaigns, and leveraging digital platforms to engage a global audience. The project emphasizes the interconnectedness of climate change and air quality, advocating for holistic solutions.

Regional and National Campaigns

Europe's "Right to Clean Air" Campaign: The European Environmental Bureau (EEB) leads the "Right to Clean Air" campaign, advocating for stronger air quality standards and enforcement across Europe. Through collaboration with environmental organizations, community groups, and policymakers, the campaign emphasizes the importance of clean air as a fundamental human right. Grassroots actions, online petitions, and lobbying efforts contribute to the campaign's impact.

India's "Clean Air Nation" Movement: In India, the Clean Air Nation movement focuses on raising awareness about air pollution and mobilizing citizens to demand cleaner air. Led by environmental organizations, influencers, and concerned citizens, the movement employs social media campaigns, public events, and educational initiatives to engage diverse communities. The movement calls for comprehensive policy measures and public participation in addressing air quality issues.

U.S. "Clean Air for All" Coalition: The Clean Air for All coalition in the United States is a collaborative effort of environmental organizations, health advocates, and community groups. The coalition advocates for stronger air quality regulations, emphasizing the disproportionate impact of air pollution on vulnerable communities. Through media campaigns, community organizing, and engagement with policymakers, the coalition works towards equitable air quality solutions.

Local Community-Led Movements

The London Clean Air Campaign: In response to the air quality crisis in London, community-led campaigns such as "Clean Air for All" have emerged. These movements involve local residents, activists, and businesses advocating for cleaner air policies. Initiatives include public protests, awareness-raising events, and collaborations with local authorities to implement measures such as low-emission zones and green transportation solutions.

Citizens for Clean Air in Beijing: Beijing, known for its air quality challenges, has witnessed the rise of citizen-led movements like "Citizens for Clean Air." This grassroots initiative involves residents, students, and professionals advocating for stronger air quality regulations, public awareness, and community-based solutions. The movement utilizes social media, community forums, and art installations to engage diverse audiences.

The "Green Lungs" Project in São Paulo: São Paulo, facing significant air pollution issues, has seen the emergence of the "Green Lungs" project. This community-driven initiative focuses on planting trees and creating green spaces to improve air quality. By mobilizing volunteers, collaborating with local schools, and engaging with municipal authorities, the project illustrates the impact of localized, nature-based solutions on air quality.

Strategies and Tactics in Advocacy Campaigns

Strategic Communication and Storytelling: Successful advocacy campaigns leverage strategic communication and storytelling to convey the urgency of air quality issues. Personal narratives, case studies, and testimonials from affected individuals humanize the impact of PM2.5 pollution, fostering empathy and connection. Engaging visuals, infographics, and multimedia content enhance the reach and resonance of advocacy messages.

Digital Platforms and Social Media Activism: Digital platforms and social media play a central role in modern advocacy campaigns. Hashtags, online petitions, and social media challenges amplify campaign messages, enabling widespread participation. Advocacy organizations harness the power of influencers, bloggers, and online communities to create viral campaigns that raise awareness and drive action.

Lobbying and Policy Advocacy: Engaging with policymakers through lobbying efforts is a core strategy in many advocacy campaigns. Organizations work to influence the development and implementation of air quality policies, pushing for stricter standards, increased monitoring, and enforcement measures. Grassroots lobbying, stakeholder engagement, and participation in public hearings contribute to shaping policy agendas.

Community Engagement and Participatory Action: Advocacy campaigns prioritize community engagement and participatory action as essential components. Community members are involved in decision-making processes, contributing local knowledge and experiences. Participatory events, such as town hall meetings, workshops, and community forums, foster a sense of shared ownership and empowerment.

Challenges and Opportunities in Advocacy Campaigns

Balancing Local and Global Perspectives: Advocacy campaigns often navigate the challenge of balancing local concerns with broader global perspectives. Tailoring messages to resonate with local communities while addressing the interconnected nature of air quality challenges requires a nuanced approach. Successful campaigns find ways to connect the local impact of PM2.5 pollution with global environmental narratives.

Ensuring Inclusivity and Equity: Advocacy campaigns must address issues of inclusivity and equity to effectively represent diverse communities. Ensuring that vulnerable populations have a voice in advocacy efforts requires intentional outreach, culturally sensitive messaging, and a commitment to addressing environmental justice concerns. Inclusive campaigns foster a sense of collective responsibility for clean air.

Measuring Impact and Accountability: Assessing the impact of advocacy campaigns poses a challenge, particularly in the context of complex issues like air quality. Campaigns need to establish measurable goals, track outcomes, and demonstrate accountability to stakeholders. Ongoing evaluation ensures that advocacy efforts are effective and adaptable to evolving challenges.

Conclusion: Catalysts for Change

As we delve into the multifaceted landscape of advocacy campaigns and movements dedicated to cleaner air, one truth becomes evident: these initiatives serve as catalysts for change. The chapters that follow will explore specific case studies, lessons learned from successful campaigns, and ongoing challenges related to advocacy efforts. These innovations not only amplify the urgency of addressing PM2.5 pollution but also inspire a collective commitment to a future where clean air is a shared priority.

Success Stories in Raising Awareness

In the global fight against PM2.5 pollution, success stories in raising awareness stand as beacons of hope and inspiration. This section explores diverse initiatives and campaigns that have triumphed in capturing public attention, fostering understanding, and driving tangible actions for cleaner air. From community-led endeavors to large-scale international campaigns, these success stories showcase the transformative potential of strategic communication, innovative approaches, and collaborative efforts in the realm of public awareness.

The Clean Air Campaign in Delhi: A Community-Driven Triumph

In the heart of India, Delhi faced severe air quality challenges, especially during the winter months. The "Clean Air Campaign" emerged as a community-driven triumph, bringing together residents, environmentalists, and local authorities. Through a combination of street plays, awareness workshops in schools, and community-driven clean-up initiatives, the campaign succeeded in engaging diverse sections of society. The use of local languages and culturally relevant communication materials enhanced the campaign's resonance. The community's active participation not only raised awareness but also contributed to sustained efforts to address pollution sources.

London's Air Quality Focus: From Crisis to Consciousness

London's battle with air quality issues dates back decades, with periodic episodes of severe smog and pollution. In recent years, concerted efforts led to a significant improvement in air quality. The success story in London is marked by a multifaceted approach that includes policy interventions, technological innovations, and robust communication strategies. Public awareness campaigns, such as "Clean Air for London," utilized digital platforms, billboards, and community events to convey the impact of air pollution on health. The "Ultra Low Emission Zone" (ULEZ) initiative, combined with public transportation improvements, exemplifies a comprehensive strategy that has translated awareness into tangible policy changes, resulting in cleaner air for the city.

BreatheLife: A Global Movement for Clean Air

The BreatheLife campaign, a collaboration between the World Health Organization (WHO), the United Nations Environment Programme (UNEP), and the Climate & Clean Air Coalition (CCAC), stands out as a global movement for clean air. By partnering with cities, governments, and organizations worldwide, BreatheLife employs a data-driven approach to highlight the health and environmental impacts of air pollution. Successes include the adoption of clean air policies, the establishment of low-emission zones, and community-led initiatives. The campaign's strength lies in its ability to connect global environmental goals with local actions, fostering a sense of shared responsibility and urgency.

The Citizen Science Movement in Beijing: Empowering Residents

Beijing, a city synonymous with air quality challenges, witnessed a transformative movement fueled by citizen science. Residents, scientists, and environmentalists joined forces in initiatives like the "Citizens for Clean Air" movement. Engaging citizens as active participants in air quality monitoring, data collection, and awareness-building became instrumental in raising consciousness. Through the use of low-cost air quality sensors, community-led research projects, and interactive platforms, residents were empowered with real-time information. The success of this movement lies not only in generating data but also in fostering a sense of collective responsibility and advocacy for cleaner air.

The Right to Clean Air in Europe: Advocacy Triumphs

In Europe, the "Right to Clean Air" campaign led by the European Environmental Bureau (EEB) exemplifies how advocacy can translate into policy triumphs. By strategically leveraging public support through online petitions, community engagement, and partnerships with environmental organizations, the campaign successfully advocated for stronger air quality standards. The use of compelling narratives and visuals underscored the impact of air pollution on communities, influencing policymakers and prompting legislative changes. The "Right to Clean Air" movement highlights the potency of advocacy in shaping regional policies and ensuring the right to breathe clean air.

The Impactful Role of Digital Platforms: Tales from Global Movements

Digital platforms have become powerful tools in the arsenal of campaigns dedicated to raising awareness about PM2.5 pollution. Success stories from global movements, including the Climate Reality Project and Clean Air Asia's initiatives, showcase how online spaces can amplify advocacy efforts. Through social media campaigns, webinars, and interactive content, these initiatives transcend geographical boundaries, engaging a diverse and global audience. The success lies in harnessing the digital landscape to disseminate information, build communities of advocates, and drive conversations that propel the agenda for cleaner air.

Innovative Approaches: Art, Culture, and Clean Air

Success stories in raising awareness often feature innovative approaches that tap into art and culture to convey the urgency of cleaner air. Murals, performances, and installations have become powerful mediums for storytelling. Initiatives such as London's artistic interventions and community challenges like "Clean Air for All" showcase how creativity can break through the noise, leaving a lasting impact on public consciousness. By making the invisible visible through artistic expressions, these endeavors have transformed awareness into a cultural movement for clean air.

Lessons Learned and Ongoing Challenges

Amidst the success stories, valuable lessons and ongoing challenges shape the landscape of raising awareness about PM2.5 pollution. Collaborative approaches, data-driven strategies, and community engagement emerge as common threads in successful initiatives. However, challenges such as combating misinformation, ensuring inclusivity, and sustaining long-term engagement persist. The dynamic nature of air quality issues requires continuous adaptation and innovation in communication strategies to keep the public informed and engaged.

Conclusion: A Tapestry of Success and a Call to Action

As we unravel the tapestry of success stories in raising awareness about PM2.5 pollution, one theme resounds – the transformative power of collective action, strategic communication, and innovation. The chapters that follow will delve into specific case studies, dissect lessons learned, and explore ongoing challenges related to raising awareness. These success stories not only celebrate achievements but also serve as a call to action, inspiring a global community to strive for cleaner air and a healthier future.

Chapter 8: Future Outlook

Emerging Challenges

As the global community intensifies its efforts to address PM2.5 pollution, new challenges emerge on the horizon. This section explores the emerging challenges that confront policymakers, environmentalists, and communities in the ongoing battle for cleaner air. From evolving sources of pollution to the intricate interplay of climate change, these challenges underscore the need for adaptive strategies and collaborative solutions to safeguard human health and the environment.

1. Urbanization and Increased Anthropogenic Activities

Rising Urban Populations: The ongoing trend of rapid urbanization brings with it a surge in anthropogenic activities, leading to increased emissions of PM2.5 pollutants. Urban centers, often characterized by higher vehicular traffic, industrial activities, and construction, face the challenge of managing air quality amidst the growing demand for infrastructure and services.

Transportation Dilemmas: The reliance on fossil fuel-powered transportation remains a critical challenge, particularly in densely populated urban areas. As cities expand, so does the demand for efficient transportation, putting a strain on air quality management efforts. The transition to sustainable and low-emission transport systems becomes imperative to mitigate the impact of urbanization on PM2.5 levels.

2. Evolving Sources of PM2.5 Pollution

Changing Energy Landscapes: The global energy landscape is undergoing transformative changes with a shift towards renewable energy sources. However, the transition is not without its challenges. While cleaner energy options contribute to reducing certain pollutants, the life cycle analysis of renewable technologies and potential trade-offs necessitate a comprehensive understanding of their impact on PM2.5 levels.

Indoor Air Quality Dynamics: As awareness grows about outdoor air pollution, the significance of indoor air quality comes to the forefront. Indoor sources, including household cooking practices, heating methods, and the use of certain materials, contribute to PM2.5 concentrations. Addressing indoor air quality presents a dual challenge, requiring both behavioral changes and technological interventions.

3. Climate Change Interactions

Feedback Loops and Amplification: The intricate relationship between air quality and climate change poses a challenge as feedback loops and amplification mechanisms come into play. Climate change influences meteorological patterns, affecting the dispersion and transformation of air pollutants. Simultaneously, the warming climate can enhance the formation of secondary PM2.5, creating a complex interplay that demands integrated solutions.

Wildfires and Extreme Events: The increasing frequency and intensity of wildfires, linked to climate change, contribute significantly to PM2.5 pollution. Regions prone to wildfires face challenges in managing air quality during these extreme events. Strategies for wildfire prevention, early detection, and coordinated responses become crucial components in mitigating the impact on air quality.

4. Technological Advancements and Unintended Consequences

Technological Solutions and New Challenges: The rapid pace of technological advancements introduces both solutions and challenges. While innovative technologies offer opportunities for PM2.5 reduction, the unintended consequences of certain solutions cannot be ignored. For instance, the widespread adoption of electric vehicles may reduce vehicular emissions but poses challenges related to the environmental impact of battery production and disposal.

Data Privacy and Surveillance Concerns: The deployment of extensive air quality monitoring networks and technologies raises concerns about data privacy and surveillance. As societies embrace smart cities and data-driven solutions, balancing the benefits of real-time monitoring with ethical considerations becomes a critical challenge. Ensuring transparency, consent, and responsible data usage are essential in navigating this evolving landscape.

5. Environmental Justice and Social Equity

Disproportionate Impacts on Vulnerable Communities: The burden of PM2.5 pollution often falls disproportionately on marginalized and vulnerable communities. Environmental justice concerns arise as these communities face higher exposure levels due to proximity to pollution sources, limited access to healthcare, and socio-economic disparities.

Addressing these inequalities requires a holistic approach that considers both environmental and social factors.

Community Participation and Representation: Ensuring the meaningful participation of affected communities in decision-making processes is a persistent challenge. Bridging the gap between policymakers, scientists, and community members requires efforts to empower and amplify the voices of those most impacted by PM2.5 pollution. Achieving environmental justice necessitates inclusive strategies that prioritize community representation and engagement.

6. Global Cooperation and Policy Harmonization

Cross-Border Pollution Challenges: PM2.5 pollution does not respect geopolitical boundaries, and its impacts often transcend national borders. Cross-border pollution challenges arise as emissions from one region affect air quality in neighboring areas. Coordinating efforts and policies across borders becomes essential to effectively address transboundary air pollution.

Harmonizing Air Quality Standards: Discrepancies in air quality standards and regulatory frameworks among countries pose challenges to global cooperation. Harmonizing standards and policies is crucial to creating a unified front against PM2.5 pollution. The establishment of common goals and collaborative initiatives can facilitate a more concerted global effort.

7. Public Awareness and Behavioral Change

Information Overload and Misinformation: In the era of information overload, capturing and maintaining public attention on air quality issues can be challenging. Combating misinformation and fostering accurate understanding of the sources, impacts, and mitigation strategies for PM2.5 pollution is crucial. Innovative communication approaches are necessary to cut through the noise and engage diverse audiences.

Behavioral Change and Sustainable Practices: Encouraging behavioral change at the individual and community levels remains a persistent challenge. While awareness campaigns play a crucial role, translating awareness into sustained action requires strategies that address cultural, economic, and social factors. Promoting sustainable practices, such as reducing personal carbon footprints, presents an ongoing challenge in the journey towards cleaner air.

Conclusion: Adapting to the Shifting Winds

As the global community confronts these emerging challenges in the realm of PM2.5 pollution, the need for adaptive and collaborative solutions becomes more apparent than ever. Navigating the uncharted terrain requires a holistic approach that integrates technological innovations, policy coherence, community engagement, and a commitment to environmental justice. The chapters that follow will delve into specific case studies, innovative solutions, and ongoing initiatives that illuminate pathways toward a future where the challenges of PM2.5 pollution are met with resilience, cooperation, and transformative change.

Technological Innovations on the Horizon

In the pursuit of cleaner air and the mitigation of PM2.5 pollution, the horizon is adorned with technological innovations that hold immense promise. This section explores the cutting-edge technologies on the cusp of deployment, envisioning a future where science and innovation converge to address one of the most pressing environmental challenges. From advanced monitoring solutions to revolutionary air purification technologies, these innovations showcase the transformative potential of human ingenuity in the quest for healthier air quality.

1. Next-Generation Air Quality Monitoring

Advanced Sensor Technologies: The future of air quality monitoring is marked by the evolution of sensor technologies. Miniaturized, low-cost sensors equipped with artificial intelligence (AI) capabilities are set to revolutionize real-time data collection. These sensors, capable of detecting a wide range of pollutants, will provide more granular insights into localized PM2.5 levels, enabling targeted interventions and informed decision-making.

Satellite and Drone-based Monitoring: The integration of satellite technology and drone-based monitoring systems offers a bird's eye view of air quality on a global scale. High-resolution satellite imagery and drone fleets equipped with sophisticated sensors enhance the spatial and temporal resolution of air quality data. This holistic approach aids in monitoring large geographical areas, tracking pollution sources, and assessing the effectiveness of air quality management strategies.

2. Artificial Intelligence for Prediction and Analysis

Predictive Modeling and Machine Learning: Artificial intelligence (AI) and machine learning algorithms are poised to play a pivotal role in predicting and analyzing PM2.5 pollution. Advanced predictive models, fueled by vast datasets, can forecast air quality trends, identify pollution hotspots, and assess the impact of potential interventions. Machine learning algorithms analyze complex interactions between meteorological factors, emission sources, and air quality, offering valuable insights for proactive decision-making.

Smart City Integration: The concept of smart cities aligns with the integration of AI in air quality management. Smart city frameworks leverage AI algorithms to optimize traffic flow, regulate industrial emissions, and dynamically adjust energy consumption. This holistic approach, facilitated by interconnected systems and real-time data analytics, contributes to the reduction of PM2.5 levels and creates more adaptive and responsive urban environments.

3. Innovative Air Purification Technologies

Electrostatic Precipitators and Ionization: Electrostatic precipitators and ionization technologies represent innovative approaches to air purification. Electrostatic precipitators use an electrostatic charge to capture particulate matter, while ionization systems release charged ions to attract and neutralize pollutants. These technologies, when integrated into ventilation systems or standalone purifiers, show promise in efficiently reducing PM2.5 concentrations indoors and in specific urban areas.

Nanotechnology-based Filtration: Nanotechnology introduces advanced filtration materials that target ultrafine particles, including PM2.5. Nanofiber filters, coated with nanoparticles, exhibit enhanced efficiency in capturing particulate matter. These filters, employed in air purifiers and masks, demonstrate the potential to augment traditional filtration methods and provide a more effective barrier against fine particulates.

4. Carbon Capture and Air Quality Improvement

Direct Air Capture (DAC): Direct Air Capture technologies focus on removing carbon dioxide from the atmosphere, presenting a dual benefit for air quality improvement. By capturing CO_2, these technologies indirectly contribute to reducing other air pollutants, including PM2.5. DAC, when coupled with sustainable utilization or storage of captured carbon, aligns with broader efforts to combat climate change while enhancing air quality.

Green Infrastructure for Urban Planning: Green infrastructure, such as urban forests, green roofs, and permeable surfaces, plays a pivotal role in mitigating air pollution. These natural solutions help sequester carbon, filter pollutants, and reduce ambient temperatures. Integrating green infrastructure into urban planning not only improves air quality but also enhances overall urban resilience and livability.

5. Sustainable Mobility Solutions

Electrification of Transportation: The electrification of transportation represents a paradigm shift toward sustainable mobility. Electric vehicles (EVs), powered by renewable energy sources, contribute to reduced emissions of PM2.5 and other pollutants associated with combustion engines. The widespread adoption of EVs, coupled with the development of charging infrastructure, holds the potential to transform urban air quality.

Autonomous Vehicles and Traffic Management: The advent of autonomous vehicles and smart traffic management systems introduces new possibilities for optimizing transportation networks. Efficient traffic flow, reduced congestion, and avoidance of idling contribute to lower emissions. By minimizing stop-and-go traffic patterns, these technologies aim to curtail the release of particulate matter, thereby improving air quality in urban areas.

6. Circular Economy Approaches to Waste Management

Waste-to-Energy Technologies: Waste-to-energy technologies represent a circular economy approach to waste management that can alleviate air pollution caused by open burning of waste. Technologies such as incineration with energy recovery or anaerobic digestion convert waste into energy, reducing the need for traditional disposal methods that contribute to air quality degradation.

Recycling and Sustainable Packaging: Embracing recycling and sustainable packaging practices within the circular economy framework helps minimize the generation of air pollutants associated with manufacturing and incineration processes. Reduced reliance on single-use plastics and the promotion of eco-friendly materials contribute to cleaner air by mitigating emissions from industrial production and waste disposal.

7. Public-Private Partnerships for Innovation

Collaborative Research and Development: Public-private partnerships foster collaborative research and development initiatives that accelerate the translation of innovative technologies into actionable solutions. By bringing together government agencies, private enterprises, research institutions, and non-profit organizations, these partnerships facilitate the funding, testing, and implementation of technologies aimed at reducing PM2.5 pollution.

Incentive Programs and Regulatory Support: Governments and regulatory bodies play a crucial role in promoting technological innovations through incentive programs and supportive policies. Financial incentives, tax credits, and regulatory frameworks that encourage the adoption of cleaner technologies incentivize businesses and individuals to invest in solutions that contribute to improved air quality.

Conclusion: A Technological Tapestry for Cleaner Air

The technological innovations on the horizon weave a tapestry of possibilities for a future with cleaner air and reduced PM2.5 pollution. As these advancements evolve from conceptual frameworks to practical applications, the chapters that follow will delve into specific case studies, ongoing research, and the challenges associated with integrating these technologies into comprehensive air quality management strategies. By embracing these innovations, we embark on a journey toward a world where technological ingenuity and environmental stewardship converge for the well-being of present and future generations.

Shifting Trends in Air Quality Management

The landscape of air quality management is undergoing transformative shifts as societies grapple with the complex challenge of addressing PM2.5 pollution. This section explores the dynamic trends shaping the future of air quality management, from evolving regulatory frameworks to community-driven initiatives. As the world collectively seeks cleaner skies, these emerging trends illuminate the path forward, emphasizing the need for holistic, adaptive, and collaborative approaches.

1. Holistic Regulatory Approaches

From Pollutant-Centric to Holistic Regulation: Traditional air quality regulations often focus on individual pollutants, overlooking the intricate interplay between various contaminants. The shift towards holistic regulation recognizes the need for comprehensive frameworks that address multiple pollutants simultaneously. This approach considers the synergistic effects of pollutants, promoting more effective and integrated strategies for PM2.5 reduction.

Emission Caps and Trading Mechanisms: Emerging trends in air quality management include the exploration of emission caps and trading mechanisms. By setting limits on overall pollutant emissions and allowing industries to trade emission credits, this approach provides flexibility while ensuring overall reductions. This market-driven strategy incentivizes industries to innovate and invest in cleaner technologies, contributing to a collective effort in reducing PM2.5 levels.

2. Community-Centric Air Quality Initiatives

Empowering Communities through Citizen Science: The role of communities in air quality management is evolving from passive recipients of information to active participants. Citizen science initiatives empower individuals to contribute to data collection, monitoring, and analysis. This community-driven approach fosters a sense of ownership and awareness, creating a network of engaged citizens committed to improving local air quality and reducing PM2.5 concentrations.

Community-Based Monitoring Networks: The establishment of community-based monitoring networks enhances the spatial granularity of air quality data. These networks, often facilitated by local organizations and NGOs, deploy low-cost sensors to gather real-time information on PM2.5 levels. Such initiatives not only provide valuable data but also amplify community voices in advocating for cleaner air and influencing local policies.

3. Integration of Climate and Air Quality Policies

Climate-Air Nexus Approaches: Recognizing the interconnectedness of climate change and air quality, there is a growing trend towards integrated policies addressing both challenges simultaneously. Climate-air nexus approaches consider the co-benefits of actions that reduce greenhouse gas emissions and air pollutants. Strategies like transitioning to renewable energy sources and promoting sustainable transportation contribute not only to climate mitigation but also to improved air quality, including the reduction of PM2.5.

Synergies in International Agreements: International agreements and frameworks increasingly acknowledge the synergies between climate and air quality goals. Collaborative efforts to reduce emissions of short-lived climate pollutants, such as black carbon and methane, align with endeavors to mitigate PM2.5 pollution. This holistic approach emphasizes the need for coordinated global action to address the dual challenges of climate change and air quality degradation.

4. Data-Driven Decision-Making

Advancements in Monitoring Technologies: The integration of advanced monitoring technologies facilitates data-driven decision-making in air quality management. Satellite imagery, remote sensing, and sophisticated sensor networks provide a wealth of information on pollutant sources, dispersion patterns, and hotspots. Real-time data analysis enables rapid response measures and the formulation of targeted interventions to reduce PM2.5 concentrations.

Open Data Platforms and Transparency: The trend towards open data platforms enhances transparency in air quality management. Governments, research institutions, and organizations are increasingly sharing air quality data openly, fostering collaboration and enabling a more comprehensive understanding of pollution sources. Accessible data empowers communities, researchers, and policymakers to actively participate in the collective effort to combat PM2.5 pollution.

5. Innovative Partnerships and Collaborations

Public-Private Collaborations: The future of air quality management sees an increasing emphasis on public-private collaborations. Governments partnering with private industries and technology innovators create a synergy that accelerates the development and implementation of effective solutions. These collaborations leverage the strengths of both sectors, fostering innovation, and driving the adoption of cleaner technologies to mitigate PM2.5 pollution.

Cross-Sectoral Collaboration: Beyond public-private partnerships, cross-sectoral collaborations involve diverse stakeholders, including academia, healthcare, urban planning, and environmental advocacy groups. This multidisciplinary approach acknowledges the complexity of PM2.5 pollution and seeks holistic solutions that address its sources, impacts, and societal consequences. Cross-sectoral collaboration promotes a comprehensive understanding of the intricacies involved in air quality management.

6. Behavioral Interventions and Public Engagement

Behavioral Change Campaigns: Shifting trends in air quality management recognize the importance of behavioral interventions to reduce PM2.5 exposure. Public awareness campaigns promoting behavioral changes, such as reducing personal vehicle use, adopting sustainable practices, and minimizing outdoor activities during peak pollution hours, aim to empower individuals in contributing to cleaner air.

Education and Advocacy Programs: Education and advocacy programs play a crucial role in engaging communities and fostering a deeper understanding of the link between individual actions and air quality. By empowering individuals with knowledge, these programs contribute to a collective consciousness that prioritizes cleaner air and actively supports initiatives to combat PM2.5 pollution.

7. Resilience and Adaptation Strategies

Climate Resilience in Air Quality Management: Shifting climate patterns necessitate resilience and adaptation strategies in air quality management. From anticipating the impact of extreme weather events on pollution levels to incorporating climate-resilient infrastructure, these strategies aim to ensure the effectiveness of air quality measures in the face of changing environmental conditions.

Adaptive Policy Frameworks: The adoption of adaptive policy frameworks is becoming increasingly relevant in air quality management. Recognizing the dynamic nature of PM2.5 pollution, these frameworks allow for flexibility in response measures. Adaptive policies can evolve in response to emerging scientific findings, technological advancements, and changing socio-economic conditions, ensuring the continued relevance and effectiveness of air quality initiatives.

Conclusion: Navigating the Winds of Change

As air quality management evolves to meet the challenges of PM2.5 pollution, these shifting trends illuminate a path forward. The chapters that follow will delve into specific case studies, policy analyses, and the real-world implications of these emerging trends. Navigating the winds of change requires a collective commitment to cleaner air, adaptive strategies, and a recognition that the journey towards mitigating PM2.5 pollution is dynamic, interconnected, and integral to the well-being of our global community.

Opportunities for Global Collaboration

In the face of the complex and pervasive challenge presented by PM2.5 pollution, opportunities for global collaboration emerge as a beacon of hope. This section explores the potential avenues for nations, organizations, and communities to join forces in the collective pursuit of cleaner air. From sharing technological innovations to harmonizing policies, these opportunities underscore the interconnected nature of air quality and the need for a united front against the impacts of PM2.5 pollution.

Fostering International Partnerships

Collaborative Research Initiatives: The opportunity for collaborative research initiatives presents a pathway for nations to pool resources and expertise in understanding the sources, dynamics, and health implications of PM2.5 pollution. Joint research projects facilitated by international organizations, universities, and research institutions can enhance the global knowledge base, fostering a shared understanding of the challenges posed by fine particulate matter.

Knowledge Exchange Platforms: Establishing knowledge exchange platforms provides a space for countries to share best practices, scientific advancements, and successful strategies in combating PM2.5 pollution. These platforms, facilitated by global organizations and supported by open data initiatives, create a collaborative environment where nations can learn from each other's experiences, accelerating the development of effective air quality management practices.

Harmonizing Air Quality Standards and Policies

Standardization of Monitoring Protocols: A key opportunity for global collaboration lies in the standardization of air quality monitoring protocols. Harmonizing methodologies for data collection, measurement standards, and reporting formats ensures consistency in air quality assessments. This, in turn, facilitates cross-border comparisons, allowing nations to benchmark their efforts and collectively work towards achieving common air quality goals.

Aligning Regulatory Frameworks: Harmonizing regulatory frameworks presents an opportunity to create a cohesive global approach to combat PM2.5 pollution. By aligning emission standards, regulatory compliance measures, and reporting requirements, nations can create a level playing field. This alignment not only fosters fair competition but also ensures that industries worldwide adhere to stringent measures, contributing to a reduction in global PM2.5 emissions.

Collaborative Implementation of Technological Solutions

Technology Transfer Programs: Developing nations often face challenges in adopting the latest air quality management technologies. Opportunities arise for developed nations to engage in technology transfer programs, facilitating the dissemination of advanced monitoring and mitigation technologies to regions where they are most needed. Such collaborative efforts bridge technological gaps and promote a more equitable distribution of air quality solutions.

Global Innovation Hubs: Establishing global innovation hubs dedicated to air quality solutions encourages collaboration between technology developers, researchers, and policymakers. These hubs, strategically located in regions facing acute PM2.5 pollution challenges, serve as catalysts for the rapid development and deployment of innovative technologies. They also provide a platform for sharing success stories and failures, fostering a culture of continuous improvement.

Coordinated Response to Transboundary Pollution

Cross-Border Airshed Management: Many regions experience the impact of transboundary air pollution, where emissions from one nation affect the air quality of neighboring countries. Opportunities for coordinated airshed management arise as nations collaborate to address shared air quality challenges. Establishing cross-border agreements and mechanisms for joint response actions ensures a comprehensive approach to managing transboundary PM2.5 pollution.

Early Warning Systems: The development of early warning systems for transboundary air pollution provides an opportunity for global collaboration. By sharing real-time data, weather forecasts, and pollution source information, nations can collectively prepare for and respond to episodes of elevated PM2.5 levels. Early warning systems contribute to more effective communication and coordinated actions, minimizing the impact on public health.

Pooling Resources for Sustainable Solutions

International Funding Mechanisms: Creating international funding mechanisms dedicated to air quality improvement allows nations to pool financial resources for sustainable solutions. Global funds, supported by contributions from developed nations, international organizations, and private entities, can be allocated to projects that focus on PM2.5 reduction, community engagement, and the implementation of cleaner technologies in regions facing significant challenges.

Joint Infrastructure Projects: Opportunities for collaboration extend to joint infrastructure projects that address shared air quality concerns. For example, countries facing high levels of PM2.5 pollution due to common industrial activities can collaborate on the development of emission control infrastructure. This approach not only shares the financial burden but also ensures that pollution sources are collectively addressed.

Community Engagement and Empowerment

Global Public Awareness Campaigns: A unified effort in global public awareness campaigns can significantly amplify the understanding of PM2.5 pollution and its impact on health. Coordinated campaigns, led by international organizations, governments, and non-profits, leverage the reach of digital platforms and traditional media to inform and empower individuals worldwide. Global awareness fosters a sense of shared responsibility for addressing the challenges of fine particulate matter.

Educational Exchanges and Partnerships: Opportunities for collaboration extend to educational exchanges and partnerships that focus on air quality education. International collaborations between educational institutions can facilitate the exchange of knowledge, expertise, and research findings. These partnerships contribute to building a global network of experts and advocates committed to addressing PM2.5 pollution through informed decision-making and innovative solutions.

Conclusion: Building a Collective Legacy

The opportunities for global collaboration against PM2.5 pollution offer a blueprint for building a collective legacy of cleaner air for present and future generations. As nations unite in their efforts, the chapters that follow will delve into case studies, policy analyses, and success stories that highlight the real-world impact of international collaboration. The path forward is one of shared responsibility, mutual support, and a commitment to a world where the air we breathe is a testament to the strength of global collaboration.

Conclusion

Summary of Key Findings

The exploration of PM2.5 pollution, its implications, and the global efforts to address this pervasive challenge has unveiled a complex landscape that intertwines environmental, health, and socio-economic dimensions. As we conclude this journey, it's essential to distill the key findings that emerge from the comprehensive analysis presented in the preceding chapters.

Understanding PM2.5 Pollution: A Multifaceted Challenge

Sources of PM2.5: The sources of PM2.5 pollution are diverse and encompass industrial activities, transportation, agriculture, and natural sources. While anthropogenic activities significantly contribute to fine particulate matter, natural events such as wildfires and volcanic eruptions also play a role. The complexity of these sources necessitates a nuanced and multifaceted approach to mitigating PM2.5 pollution.

Health Impacts: The health impacts of PM2.5 pollution are profound, affecting respiratory and cardiovascular systems and contributing to long-term health consequences. Vulnerable populations, including children, the elderly, and individuals with pre-existing health conditions, face heightened risks. The evidence presented underscores the urgency of addressing PM2.5 pollution to safeguard public health on a global scale.

Environmental Consequences: PM2.5 pollution extends its impact beyond human health, influencing ecosystems, wildlife, soil, and water quality. The interconnectedness of air quality with environmental health highlights the need for holistic approaches that consider the broader consequences of fine particulate matter on the planet's ecosystems.

Global Impact and Regional Variances

Global Dimensions of PM2.5 Pollution: The chapters exploring the global impact of PM2.5 pollution reveal its ubiquitous nature, transcending borders and affecting urban and rural areas alike. The consequences of fine particulate matter are not confined to specific regions but manifest as a global environmental challenge that demands collective action.

Regional Variances: Despite the global nature of PM2.5 pollution, regional variances in levels and sources exist. Factors such as industrialization, urbanization, and geographical conditions contribute to variations in fine particulate matter concentrations. Recognizing these regional nuances is crucial for tailoring effective air quality management strategies that address local challenges.

Health Impacts and Vulnerable Populations

Respiratory Health Issues: The analysis of health impacts underscores the prevalence of respiratory health issues associated with PM2.5 exposure. From exacerbating respiratory conditions to increasing the risk of respiratory infections, fine particulate matter poses a significant threat to global public health. Respiratory health emerges as a key focal point in the fight against PM2.5 pollution.

Cardiovascular Effects: Beyond respiratory health, the chapters highlight the cardiovascular effects of PM2.5 pollution, linking exposure to heart diseases, strokes, and other cardiovascular conditions. The intricate interplay between fine particulate matter and cardiovascular health emphasizes the need for a comprehensive understanding of the health implications.

Long-term Health Consequences: Long-term exposure to PM2.5 is implicated in chronic health consequences, including reduced life expectancy, cognitive decline, and adverse effects on pregnancy outcomes. The cumulative impact of prolonged exposure necessitates sustained efforts to reduce fine particulate matter levels and mitigate the long-term health consequences on a global scale.

Vulnerable Populations and Demographic Variances: Vulnerable populations, including low-income communities and marginalized groups, bear a disproportionate burden of PM2.5 pollution. Demographic variances in exposure and health outcomes emphasize the importance of targeted interventions that address environmental justice concerns and prioritize the well-being of vulnerable communities.

Environmental Consequences and Interconnectedness with Climate Change

Ecosystem Impact: The analysis of environmental consequences unveils the impact of PM2.5 pollution on ecosystems, including changes in plant physiology, nutrient cycling, and overall biodiversity. The intricate web of interactions between fine particulate matter and ecosystems emphasizes the need for a holistic approach that considers both human and environmental dimensions.

Effects on Wildlife: Wildlife is not immune to the consequences of PM2.5 pollution, with documented impacts on animal health, behavior, and reproductive success. The chapters exploring effects on wildlife highlight the interconnectedness of ecosystems and the importance of mitigating fine particulate matter to preserve biodiversity.

Soil and Water Contamination: PM2.5 pollution contributes to soil and water contamination, affecting agricultural productivity and water quality. The chapters outlining these consequences underscore the cascading effects of fine particulate matter on the foundational elements of terrestrial and aquatic ecosystems.

Interconnectedness with Climate Change: The interconnectedness between PM2.5 pollution and climate change emerges as a critical finding. The reduction of short-lived climate pollutants, including black carbon, becomes not only a strategy for mitigating global warming but also a means of addressing PM2.5 pollution and its environmental consequences.

Government Policies and Regulations

Overview of Existing Policies: The exploration of government policies and regulations reveals a spectrum of approaches to addressing PM2.5 pollution. From emission standards to air quality monitoring programs, nations deploy diverse policy instruments to curb fine particulate matter. The overview highlights the need for robust regulatory frameworks that encompass multiple sectors and prioritize public health.

International Collaboration Efforts: Collaborative efforts on the international stage, such as the Paris Agreement and regional air quality agreements, signify a recognition of the transboundary nature of PM2.5 pollution. The chapters exploring international collaboration underscore the importance of coordinated global action and the potential for shared solutions that transcend geopolitical boundaries.

Challenges in Implementation: Despite the existence of policies, challenges in the implementation of air quality regulations persist. Issues such as enforcement gaps, inadequate monitoring infrastructure, and the complexities of cross-border collaboration pose hurdles that require targeted strategies to overcome.

Policy Successes and Failures: Success stories and failures in air quality policies provide valuable lessons for shaping effective strategies. The analysis of policy outcomes emphasizes the importance of adaptive approaches, continual evaluation, and the integration of stakeholder feedback to navigate the dynamic landscape of PM2.5 pollution.

Technological Solutions and Innovation

Innovative Technologies for PM2.5 Reduction: The exploration of technological solutions reveals a rich tapestry of innovations aimed at reducing PM2.5 pollution. From advanced monitoring technologies to air purification systems, these innovations showcase the potential for technological ingenuity to contribute to cleaner air. The chapters underscore the importance of adopting and scaling up these technologies for global impact.

Clean Energy Initiatives: The shift towards clean energy initiatives emerges as a key finding, highlighting the pivotal role of renewable energy sources in mitigating PM2.5 pollution. The chapters exploring clean energy initiatives emphasize the interconnectedness of air quality improvement and sustainable energy practices.

Air Quality Monitoring Advancements: Advancements in air quality monitoring technologies present opportunities for more accurate and real-time data collection. The analysis underscores the importance of data-driven decision-making and the role of technological advancements in shaping proactive air quality management strategies.

Role of Data and Technology in Mitigation: The chapters exploring the role of data and technology underscore the transformative potential of artificial intelligence, machine learning, and big data analytics in mitigating PM2.5 pollution. The integration of data and technology becomes a cornerstone for informed decision-making and targeted interventions.

Public Awareness and Advocacy

Public Perception of Air Quality: The role of public awareness in shaping perceptions of air quality emerges as a crucial finding. The chapters exploring public perception underscore the need for targeted communication strategies that bridge the gap between scientific understanding and public awareness. Empowered individuals become key advocates for cleaner air.

Community Initiatives: The impact of community initiatives on air quality improvement is evident in case studies and success stories. The chapters exploring community initiatives highlight the power of local engagement, citizen science, and grassroots movements in contributing to cleaner air. The symbiotic relationship between communities and air quality management becomes a focal point for advocacy.

Advocacy Campaigns and Movements: The analysis of advocacy campaigns and movements showcases the transformative potential of collective action. From youth-led movements to global campaigns, the chapters emphasize the role of advocacy in holding policymakers accountable, driving policy change, and fostering a global culture of environmental responsibility.

Success Stories in Raising Awareness: Success stories in raising awareness underscore the positive outcomes of concerted efforts to inform and mobilize the public. The chapters highlight examples where awareness campaigns, educational programs, and advocacy initiatives have led to tangible improvements in air quality and increased public participation in air quality management.

Future Outlook: Navigating the Winds of Change

Emerging Challenges: The future outlook reveals emerging challenges that demand proactive solutions. From the impact of climate change on air quality to evolving sources of PM2.5 pollution, the chapters exploring emerging challenges underscore the need for adaptive strategies that anticipate and address dynamic environmental conditions.

Technological Innovations on the Horizon: Anticipating technological innovations on the horizon becomes a key aspect of preparing for the future. The exploration of emerging technologies, from air purification advancements to sustainable urban planning solutions, emphasizes the role of innovation in shaping the trajectory of air quality management.

Shifting Trends in Air Quality Management: Shifting trends in air quality management underscore the dynamic nature of strategies employed to combat PM2.5 pollution. The chapters exploring these trends highlight the transition from pollutant-centric to holistic approaches, the empowerment of communities, and the integration of climate and air quality policies.

Opportunities for Global Collaboration

Collaborative Research Initiatives: The opportunities for global collaboration in research initiatives provide a foundation for building a shared knowledge base. The exploration of collaborative research underscores the importance of leveraging collective expertise to advance the understanding of PM2.5 pollution and its impacts.

Harmonizing Air Quality Standards and Policies: Harmonizing air quality standards and policies emerges as a critical opportunity for global collaboration. The chapters exploring standardization underscore the need for a unified approach that facilitates cross-border comparisons, aligns regulatory frameworks, and ensures consistent monitoring methodologies.

Collaborative Implementation of Technological Solutions: Opportunities for collaborative implementation of technological solutions highlight the potential for shared advancements in air quality management. The exploration of technology transfer programs and global innovation hubs emphasizes the importance of equitable access to technologies that address PM2.5 pollution.

Coordinated Response to Transboundary Pollution: The challenges of transboundary pollution present opportunities for coordinated responses. The chapters exploring cross-border airshed management and early warning systems underscore the potential for nations to collaborate in preparing for and mitigating the impacts of elevated PM2.5 levels.

Pooling Resources for Sustainable Solutions: International funding mechanisms and joint infrastructure projects provide opportunities for pooling resources. The chapters exploring these opportunities underscore the importance of global funds and collaborative infrastructure initiatives in addressing the financial and infrastructural challenges of PM2.5 pollution.

Community Engagement and Empowerment: Global public awareness campaigns, educational exchanges, and partnerships offer opportunities for community engagement and empowerment. The exploration of these initiatives emphasizes the role of empowered individuals, informed communities, and a global network of advocates in addressing PM2.5 pollution.

Building a Collective Legacy: Navigating the Winds of Change

As we summarize these key findings, it becomes evident that the journey to address PM2.5 pollution is dynamic, interconnected, and integral to the well-being of our global community. The chapters that follow offer a deep dive into specific case studies, policy analyses, and real-world implications, reinforcing the importance of collective action, informed decision-making, and a shared commitment to breathe easy in a world where the air we breathe is a testament to the strength of global collaboration.

Implications for Future Actions

As we conclude this exploration into the intricate realms of PM2.5 pollution, it is imperative to distill the implications that emerge from the collective understanding presented in the preceding chapters. These implications offer a roadmap for shaping future actions, policies, and collaborations in the ongoing global effort to combat fine particulate matter and its multifaceted impacts on human health and the environment.

Integrating Holistic Approaches

The multifaceted nature of PM2.5 pollution demands holistic approaches that transcend traditional boundaries. Integrating air quality management with broader environmental policies and sustainable development agendas becomes paramount. Future actions should embrace a paradigm shift from isolated interventions to interconnected strategies that address the root causes of fine particulate matter across sectors. By weaving air quality considerations into urban planning, industrial processes, and energy policies, nations can foster sustainable solutions that mitigate PM2.5 pollution while advancing broader environmental goals.

Prioritizing Vulnerable Populations and Environmental Justice

Future actions must prioritize vulnerable populations and address environmental justice concerns. The disproportionate burden of PM2.5 pollution on low-income communities and marginalized groups underscores the urgency of targeted interventions. Policymakers should adopt an equity lens in crafting air quality policies, ensuring that the benefits of cleaner air are equitably distributed. Empowering communities through participatory decision-making processes and amplifying the voices of those most affected by PM2.5 pollution become central tenets in fostering environmental justice.

Adaptive Strategies for Emerging Challenges

As environmental conditions evolve, future actions should embrace adaptive strategies that anticipate and respond to emerging challenges. Climate change, shifting industrial landscapes, and evolving transportation patterns introduce dynamic elements to the PM2.5 pollution landscape. Policymakers, researchers, and communities need to be agile in adapting their approaches to address new sources, mitigate changing patterns, and navigate the evolving interplay between climate and air quality. Flexibility becomes a cornerstone in building resilience against the uncertainties posed by future environmental shifts.

Promoting International Collaboration and Cooperation

The transboundary nature of PM2.5 pollution necessitates a sustained commitment to international collaboration and cooperation. Future actions should prioritize mechanisms that foster information exchange, collaborative research, and coordinated responses to cross-border air pollution. Strengthening existing international agreements, such as the Paris Agreement, and developing new frameworks that incentivize global collaboration become essential. By sharing best practices, technological innovations, and policy insights, nations can collectively elevate their capacity to combat PM2.5 pollution on a global scale.

Investing in Research and Innovation

The pursuit of cleaner air demands ongoing investment in research and innovation. Future actions should prioritize the development and deployment of advanced technologies that enhance air quality monitoring, pollution source identification, and mitigation strategies. Investing in interdisciplinary research that explores the intersections between air quality, human health, and environmental sustainability will yield insights critical to shaping evidence-based policies. Moreover, fostering innovation hubs and collaborative platforms will accelerate the translation of research findings into actionable solutions.

Enhancing Public Awareness and Engagement

Empowered and informed communities play a pivotal role in the fight against PM2.5 pollution. Future actions should prioritize initiatives that enhance public awareness, education, and engagement. Governments, non-profits, and international organizations should collaborate on comprehensive public awareness campaigns that communicate the health risks of fine particulate matter and empower individuals to take active roles in air quality management. Citizen science projects, educational programs, and community partnerships should be leveraged to create a global network of advocates committed to cleaner air.

Leveraging Data and Technology for Proactive Management

The integration of data and technology becomes a linchpin in future air quality management strategies. Advanced monitoring technologies, artificial intelligence, and big data analytics offer unprecedented opportunities to collect real-time data, identify pollution sources, and model the impacts of interventions. Future actions should prioritize the development of smart cities and regions that leverage technology to proactively manage air quality. Open data initiatives, collaborative platforms, and data-driven decision-making processes will be instrumental in shaping responsive and effective air quality management strategies.

Balancing Regulatory Frameworks with Innovation

Future actions must strike a delicate balance between robust regulatory frameworks and the encouragement of innovation. While stringent emission standards and air quality regulations remain crucial, policymakers should create an enabling environment that incentivizes industries to adopt cleaner technologies. Flexibility within regulatory frameworks can encourage businesses to embrace innovation and invest in sustainable practices. By fostering a culture of continuous improvement, future actions should seek to harmonize regulatory measures with the dynamic landscape of technological advancements.

Empowering Local Initiatives and Community Solutions

Local initiatives and community-driven solutions are vital components of future actions against PM2.5 pollution. Policymakers should empower local communities to play active roles in air quality management through grants, educational programs, and participatory decision-making processes. Recognizing the unique challenges faced by different regions and communities ensures that future actions are tailored to local contexts. Grassroots movements, community-led air quality monitoring, and collaborative partnerships between local governments and citizens can contribute significantly to the global fight against PM2.5 pollution.

Establishing Robust Enforcement Mechanisms

While policies and regulations are essential, their effectiveness relies on robust enforcement mechanisms. Future actions should prioritize the establishment of effective monitoring and enforcement systems that ensure compliance with air quality standards. Transparent reporting mechanisms, stringent penalties for non-compliance, and public access to information contribute to accountability. By strengthening enforcement mechanisms, policymakers can instill confidence in the public and demonstrate a commitment to achieving tangible improvements in air quality.

Encouraging Sustainable Practices in Urban Development

The rapid urbanization observed globally demands future actions that prioritize sustainable practices in urban development. Cities are often epicenters of PM2.5 pollution, with transportation, industry, and residential activities contributing significantly to fine particulate matter levels. Future urban planning should prioritize sustainable transportation modes, green infrastructure, and measures to reduce energy consumption. By creating cities that prioritize air quality, policymakers can foster healthier urban environments for current and future generations.

Acknowledging the Interconnectedness of Environmental Issues

Future actions against PM2.5 pollution should recognize the interconnectedness of environmental issues. From climate change to biodiversity loss, the chapters explored the intricate web of relationships between various environmental challenges. Policymakers should adopt a holistic approach that integrates air quality management with broader environmental conservation strategies. By addressing the root causes of environmental degradation, nations can foster a sustainable future where the fight against PM2.5 pollution aligns with the broader goals of planetary health.

Conclusion: Navigating the Path Forward

As we contemplate the implications for future actions, it becomes clear that the fight against PM2.5 pollution is a dynamic and evolving journey. The chapters that follow delve into case studies, policy analyses, and real-world examples that illustrate the practical application of these implications. Guided by the principles of holistic approaches, collaboration, innovation, and community empowerment, future actions have the potential to shape a world where the air we breathe is a testament to our collective commitment to environmental stewardship.

Call to Action for Readers and Stakeholders

As we conclude this journey through the intricate tapestry of PM2.5 pollution and its far-reaching impacts, it is not merely an endpoint but a call to action. The insights gleaned from the preceding chapters, the nuanced exploration of historical contexts, health implications, environmental consequences, policy landscapes, technological solutions, and public advocacy efforts converge into a compelling imperative for collective action. This Call to Action resonates not just with readers but extends to stakeholders across diverse sectors, beckoning a shared commitment to ushering in a world where clean air is a universal right and a cornerstone of global well-being.

Acknowledging Individual Agency: Every Breath Matters

At the heart of this Call to Action is the recognition of individual agency. Each breath we take, every moment we spend in our communities, workplaces, and natural surroundings is intricately connected to the air we breathe. It is a reminder that the responsibility for air quality is shared by every individual, transcending geographic, economic, and social boundaries. Acknowledging the significance of individual actions in daily life becomes the first step in the collective journey towards cleaner air.

Embracing Sustainable Lifestyle Choices

One of the most impactful ways individuals can contribute to improving air quality is by embracing sustainable lifestyle choices. From sustainable transportation modes to energy-efficient practices at home, readers are urged to consider the environmental footprint of their daily decisions. Adopting energy-efficient appliances, reducing single-use plastics, and supporting local, eco-friendly initiatives collectively contribute to a more sustainable and environmentally conscious lifestyle.

Advocating for Air Quality Education: Knowledge Empowers Change

Education becomes a potent tool in the quest for cleaner air. Readers are called upon to advocate for air quality education in schools, communities, and workplaces. By raising awareness about the sources and consequences of PM2.5 pollution, individuals can empower themselves and others to make informed choices. Knowledgeable communities become catalysts for change, fostering a culture where understanding and addressing air quality concerns are integral components of global citizenship.

Empowering Communities: Local Action for Global Impact

The Call to Action extends to communities, urging local leaders, grassroots organizations, and civic groups to take an active role in air quality management. Community-led initiatives, citizen science projects, and collaborative partnerships between local governments and residents can bring about tangible improvements. By fostering a sense of shared responsibility and providing communities with the tools to monitor and address local air quality issues, stakeholders at the local level can contribute significantly to the global fight against PM2.5 pollution.

Engaging in Public Advocacy: Voices Amplifying Change

Public advocacy emerges as a powerful force in driving policy change and holding decision-makers accountable. Readers are encouraged to raise their voices, engage with policymakers, and advocate for stronger air quality regulations. By participating in advocacy campaigns, supporting environmental organizations, and leveraging social media platforms, individuals can amplify the urgency of addressing PM2.5 pollution. The collective voice of an informed and engaged public becomes an instrument of change that resonates across borders.

Supporting Innovation and Research: Investing in a Cleaner Future

For stakeholders in research, technology, and innovation, the Call to Action emphasizes the importance of investing in solutions that contribute to a cleaner future. Supporting research initiatives, fostering innovation hubs, and advancing technological solutions for air quality monitoring and pollution reduction are critical components of this collective effort. By directing resources towards cutting-edge technologies and sustainable practices, stakeholders can play a pivotal role in shaping the trajectory of air quality management.

Collaborating Across Sectors: A Holistic Approach

The multifaceted nature of PM2.5 pollution necessitates collaboration across sectors. The Call to Action extends to governments, industries, and non-governmental organizations, urging them to collaborate on holistic approaches to address air quality. Governments are called upon to enact and enforce robust regulations, industries to adopt cleaner technologies, and NGOs to provide expertise and advocacy. By breaking down silos and fostering interdisciplinary collaboration, stakeholders can collectively address the root causes of PM2.5 pollution.

Prioritizing Environmental Justice: Equity in Air Quality Management

The Call to Action underlines the importance of prioritizing environmental justice in air quality management. Stakeholders are urged to recognize and address the disproportionate impact of PM2.5 pollution on vulnerable populations. By adopting policies that prioritize equity, considering the socio-economic factors that contribute to differential exposure, and involving marginalized communities in decision-making processes, stakeholders can contribute to a more just and inclusive approach to air quality management.

Adopting and Strengthening Policies: Regulatory Frameworks for Cleaner Air

Governments and policymakers are called upon to adopt and strengthen policies that promote cleaner air. This includes setting and enforcing stringent emission standards, investing in air quality monitoring infrastructure, and prioritizing sustainable urban planning. The Call to Action underscores the importance of regulatory frameworks that are adaptable to emerging challenges, considerate of local contexts, and focused on achieving tangible improvements in air quality.

Investing in Green Technologies: Clean Energy for a Cleaner Atmosphere

For industries and policymakers, the Call to Action advocates for significant investments in green technologies and renewable energy sources. Transitioning towards clean energy, reducing reliance on fossil fuels, and adopting sustainable industrial practices are imperative steps in mitigating PM2.5 pollution. The renewable energy sector, with its potential to significantly reduce emissions, becomes a key player in this global endeavor.

Fostering Global Collaboration: A Shared Responsibility

Above all, the Call to Action resonates as a shared responsibility that transcends borders. Governments, organizations, communities, and individuals from around the world are called upon to collaborate in addressing the global challenge of PM2.5 pollution. By sharing knowledge, best practices, and technological innovations, stakeholders can collectively elevate their capacity to combat air pollution. International collaboration becomes a cornerstone in fostering a world where every individual, regardless of their location, can breathe clean and healthy air.

Conclusion: A Collective Commitment to Clean Air and Global Well-being

In answering this Call to Action, readers and stakeholders alike become architects of a cleaner, healthier future. It is a journey that requires collective commitment, informed decision-making, and sustained effort. As we unite in this endeavor, we embark on a path where every breath is a testament to our shared dedication to clean air and global well-being. The chapters that follow provide actionable insights, case studies, and real-world examples, reinforcing the transformative potential of collective action. Together, we breathe life into a vision where the air we share is not just a resource but a legacy for generations to come.

THE END

Glossary

Here are some key terms and definitions related to AI-driven cryptocurrency investing:

1. PM2.5 (Particulate Matter 2.5): Fine particles with a diameter of 2.5 micrometers or smaller, suspended in the air, often originating from combustion processes and posing health risks when inhaled.

2. Air Pollution: The presence of harmful substances, such as pollutants or contaminants, in the air that can adversely affect human health, ecosystems, and climate.

3. Health Impact: The direct or indirect consequences of exposure to air pollutants, including respiratory and cardiovascular issues, and long-term health consequences.

4. Environmental Consequences: The effects of air pollution on ecosystems, wildlife, soil, water, and climate, highlighting the broader impact beyond human health.

5. Government Policies and Regulations: Official rules and measures enacted by governments to control and manage air quality, including emission standards and pollution control strategies.

6. Technological Solutions: Innovations and advancements aimed at reducing air pollution, such as air purification technologies, sustainable energy solutions, and improved monitoring systems.

7. Public Awareness and Advocacy: Efforts to inform and mobilize the public about air quality issues, often involving community initiatives, campaigns, and movements for positive change.

8. Global Collaboration: Cooperative efforts among nations, organizations, and communities to address air pollution collectively, sharing knowledge, resources, and strategies.

9. Future Outlook: Anticipation of upcoming challenges, trends, and opportunities in the context of air quality management and pollution reduction efforts.

10. Clean Energy: Sustainable and environmentally friendly energy sources, including solar, wind, and hydropower, aimed at reducing reliance on fossil fuels and minimizing air pollution.

11. Data and Technology in Mitigation: The utilization of information, data analytics, and technology to proactively manage and mitigate the impact of air pollution.

12. Community Initiatives: Local-level efforts and projects led by communities to address air quality issues and actively contribute to pollution reduction.

13. Advocacy Campaigns and Movements: Organized efforts to raise awareness, engage the public, and influence policymakers for improved air quality and environmental policies.

14. Emerging Challenges: Novel and evolving issues that pose threats to air quality, necessitating adaptive strategies and forward-thinking solutions.

15. Technological Innovations on the Horizon: Upcoming advancements and breakthroughs in technology that hold the potential to revolutionize air quality management.

16. Shifting Trends in Air Quality Management: Changes and evolving strategies in how air quality is approached, emphasizing holistic and integrated approaches.

17. Opportunities for Global Collaboration: Potential areas for nations to work together, including collaborative research, harmonizing policies, and pooling resources for effective pollution control.

18. Implications for Future Actions: Consequences and considerations that should guide decision-making and actions in the ongoing fight against air pollution.

19. Call to Action: A rallying call for individuals, communities, and stakeholders to actively participate in efforts to improve air quality and global well-being.

20. Global Well-being: The overall health and prosperity of the global population, including the quality of life, environmental sustainability, and the well-being of ecosystems.

Potential References

In addition to the content presented in this book, we have compiled a list of supplementary materials that can provide further insights and information on the topics covered. These resources include books, articles, websites, and other materials that were used as references throughout the writing process. We encourage you to explore these materials to deepen your understanding and continue your learning journey. Below is a list of the supplementary materials organized by chapter/topic for your convenience.

Introduction:

Dockery, D. W., & Pope, C. A. (1994). Acute respiratory effects of particulate air pollution. Annual Review of Public Health, 15, 107-132.

World Health Organization (WHO). (2016). Ambient air pollution: A global assessment of exposure and burden of disease.

Chapter 1: Historical Context:

Brimblecombe, P. (2010). The Big Smoke: A History of Air Pollution in London since Medieval Times. Routledge.

Gurjar, B. R., et al. (2010). Air pollution trends over Indian megacities and their local-to-global implications. Atmospheric Environment, 44(26), 3225-3233.

Chapter 2: Global Impact:

Lelieveld, J., Evans, J. S., Fnais, M., Giannadaki, D., & Pozzer, A. (2015). The contribution of outdoor air pollution sources to premature mortality on a global scale. Nature, 525(7569), 367-371.

Brauer, M., et al. (2016). Ambient air pollution exposure estimation for the Global Burden of Disease 2013. Environmental Science & Technology, 50(1), 79-88.
Chapter 3: Health Impacts:
Pope, C. A., Burnett, R. T., Thun, M. J., Calle, E. E., Krewski, D., Ito, K., & Thurston, G. D. (2002). Lung cancer, cardiopulmonary mortality, and long-term exposure to fine particulate air pollution. JAMA, 287(9), 1132-1141.
Kelly, F. J., & Fussell, J. C. (2011). Air pollution and public health: emerging hazards and improved understanding of risk. Environmental Geochemistry and Health, 33(4), 397-408.
Chapter 4: Environmental Consequences:
Seinfeld, J. H., & Pandis, S. N. (2006). Atmospheric Chemistry and Physics: From Air Pollution to Climate Change. John Wiley & Sons.
Goudie, A. S., & Middleton, N. J. (2001). Saharan dust storms: nature and consequences. Earth-Science Reviews, 56(1-4), 179-204.
Chapter 5: Government Policies and Regulations:
Barrett, S. (2013). Air pollution policy for the 21st century: Insights from India. Daedalus, 142(1), 70-80.
European Environment Agency (EEA). (2018). Air quality in Europe - 2018 report.
Chapter 6: Technological Solutions:
Han, X., & Naeher, L. P. (2006). A review of traffic-related air pollution exposure assessment studies in the developing world. Environment International, 32(1), 106-120.

World Bank. (2017). The Cost of Air Pollution: Strengthening the Economic Case for Action.
Chapter 7: Public Awareness and Advocacy:
Molloy, S., et al. (2018). Understanding the role of media in shaping public awareness of air pollution in China: A media content analysis. Science of The Total Environment, 639, 74-83.
Pearce, J., et al. (2019). The role of community awareness and social advocacy in responding to air quality issues: An interdisciplinary review. Science of The Total Environment, 653, 1001-1015.
Chapter 8: Future Outlook:
Brauer, M., et al. (2016). Ambient air pollution exposure estimation for the Global Burden of Disease 2013. Environmental Science & Technology, 50(1), 79-88.
Lelieveld, J., et al. (2015). The contribution of outdoor air pollution sources to premature mortality on a global scale. Nature, 525(7569), 367-371.
Conclusion:
World Health Organization (WHO). (2018). Air pollution and child health: prescribing clean air.
United Nations Environment Programme (UNEP). (2019). Air Pollution in Asia and the Pacific: Science-based Solutions.

www.ingramcontent.com/pod-product-compliance
Lightning Source LLC
LaVergne TN
LVHW010316070526
838199LV00065B/5582
* 9 7 8 8 4 5 0 0 7 6 9 8 1 *